To
Joan B. Beach

An Illustrated Review of the ENDOCRINE SYSTEM

Glenn F. Bastian

HarperCollins*CollegePublishers*

Executive Editor: Bonnie Roesch
Cover Designer: Kay Petronio
Production Manager: Bob Cooper
Printer and Binder: Malloy Lithographing, Inc.
Cover Printer: The Lehigh Press, Inc.

AN ILLUSTRATED REVIEW OF THE ENDOCRINE SYSTEM

by Glenn F. Bastian

Library of Congress Cataloging-in-Publication Data
Bastian, Glenn F.
        An illustrated review of the endocrine system / Glenn
    F. Bastian.
            p.   cm.
        Includes bibliographical references.
        ISBN: 0-06-501706-4
        1. Endocrine glands—Physiology—Outlines, syllabi, etc.
    2. Endocrine glands—Atlases. I. Title.
        [DNLM: 1. Endocrine Glands—ultrastructure—atlases. 2. Endocrine Glands—
    physiology—atlases. WK 17 B326i 1993]
    QM187.B37   1993
    612.4'02'02—dc20
    DNLM/DLC
    for Library of Congress   93–28457
                                                                          CIP

94 95 96 9 8 7 6 5 4 3 2

CONTENTS

LIST OF TOPICS & ILLUSTRATIONS

Text: One page of text is devoted to each of the following topics. *Illustrations are listed in italics.*

PREFACE

An Illustrated Review of Anatomy and Physiology is a series of ten books written to help students effectively review the structure and function of the human body. Each book in the series is devoted to a different body system.

My objective in writing these books is to make very complex subjects accessible and unthreatening by presenting material in manageable size bits (one topic per page) with clear, simple illustrations to assist the many students who are primarily visual learners. Designed to supplement established texts, they may be used as a student aid to jog the memory, to quickly recall the essentials of each major topic, and to practice naming structures in preparation for exams.

INNOVATIVE FEATURES OF THE BOOK

(1) Each major topic is confined to one page of text.

A unique feature of this book is that each topic is confined to one page and the material is presented in outline form with the key terms in boldface or italic typeface. This makes it easy to scan quickly the major points of any given topic. The student can easily get an overview of the topic and then zero in on a particular point that needs clarification.

(2) Each page of text has an illustration on the facing page.

Because each page of text has its illustration on the facing page, there is no need to flip through the book looking for the illustration that is referred to in the text ("see Figure X on page xx"). The purpose of the illustration is to clarify a central idea discussed in the text. The images are simple and clear, the lines are bold, and the labels are in a large type. Each illustration deals with a well-defined concept, allowing for a more focused study.

PHYSIOLOGY TOPICS (1 text page : 1 illustration)
Each main topic in physiology is limited to one page of text with one supporting illustration on the facing page.

ANATOMY TOPICS (1 text page : several illustrations)
For complex anatomical structures a good illustration is more valuable than words. So, for topics dealing with anatomy, there are often several illustrations for one text topic.

(3) Unlabeled illustrations have been included.
In Part II, all illustrations have been repeated without their labels. This allows a student to test his or her visual knowledge of the basic concepts.

(4) A Pronunciation Guide has been included.
Phonetic spellings of unfamiliar terms are listed in a separate section, unlike other textbooks where they are usually found in the glossary or spread throughout the text. The stu-dent may use this guide for pronunciation drill or as a quick review of basic vocabulary.

(5) A glossary has been included.
Most textbooks have glossaries that include terms for all of the systems of the body. It is convenient to have all of the key terms for one system in a single glossary.

ACKNOWLEDGMENTS

I would like to thank the reviewers of the manuscript for this book who carefully critiqued the text and illustrations for their effectiveness: William Kleinelp, Middlesex County College; Pamela Monaco, Molloy College; and Robert Smith, University of Missouri, St. Louis and St. Louis Community College, Forest Park. Their help and advice are greatly appreciated. I am greatly indebted to my editor Bonnie Roesch for her willingness to try a new idea, and for her support throughout this project. I invite students and instructors to send any comments and suggestions for enhancements or changes to this book to me, in care of HarperCollins, so that future editions can continue to meet your needs.

Glenn Bastian

1 Endocrine Introduction

ENDOCRINE INTRODUCTION / Overview

Neuroendocrinology

The nervous and endocrine systems are closely related; together they regulate and coordinate many body functions. The study of their common functions is called neuroendocrinology. Nervous and endocrine responses differ in their speed, duration, and specificity.

Nervous System Responses Nervous system responses are fast : it takes only a fraction of a second for a nerve impulse to travel from the brain to a muscle or gland cell. Nervous responses are of short duration : when the neurons stops firing no more neurotransmitter is released and the actions of the effector cells return to normal. Nervous responses are highly specific : only the cells that are innervated by specific nerve fibers are affected.

Endocrine System Responses Endocrine responses are relatively slow. Endocrine gland cells release hormones that travel in the bloodstream to their target cells. It takes minutes in most instances rather than fractions of a second for hormones to be released into the extracellular fluid (ECF), diffuse into nearby capillaries, and be carried by the circulating blood throughout the body. Any cells in the body that have the proper receptors for a given hormone will be affected; these are called the *target cells*. While slower in their response, the effects of hormones last longer. Until they are enzymatically altered in the liver and excreted by the kidneys, hormones continue to affect their target cells.

Endocrine Tissue

Endocrine Glands An endocrine gland is a structure whose primary function is to secrete hormones; it consists of glandular cells that are derived from epithelial tissues. Major endocrine glands are :

(1) Adrenal Gland   (4) Pituitary Gland
(2) Parathyroid Glands   (5) Thymus
(3) Pineal Gland   (6) Thyroid Gland

Structures That Contain Endocrine Tissue Many structures of the body contain endocrine tissue (cells that secrete hormones), but they have other functions as well. These include :

(1) Heart   (5) Ovaries   (9) Small Intestine
(2) Hypothalamus   (6) Pancreas   (10) Stomach
(3) Kidneys   (7) Placenta   (11) Testes
(4) Liver   (8) Skin

Major Endocrine Functions

The endocrine system regulates a wide range of body functions that include :

(1) Reproductive Processes : development of sex organs; development of secondary sexual characteristics; production of eggs and sperm; menstrual cycle.

(2) Digestive Processes : secretion of digestive enzymes; secretion of bile; secretion of gastric acid (hydrochloric acid / HCl); secretion of bicarbonate.

(3) Blood Pressure : cardiac output (heart rate and stroke volume); blood vessel constriction; water excretion by the kidneys.

(4) Blood Plasma Concentrations : glucose; minerals (sodium, potassium, calcium, and phosphorus); gases (oxygen, carbon dioxide); blood cells (erythrocytes and leukocytes); water (osmotic pressure); hydrogen ions (regulation of pH / acidity).

(5) Immune System Responses : lymphocyte activation; inflammatory response; antibody production; fever.

(6) Metabolic Rate : rate of chemical reactions in cells; the rate that cells oxidize glucose.

(7) Growth : mitosis and differentiation of tissue cells.

(8) Stress Response

MAJOR ENDOCRINE GLANDS

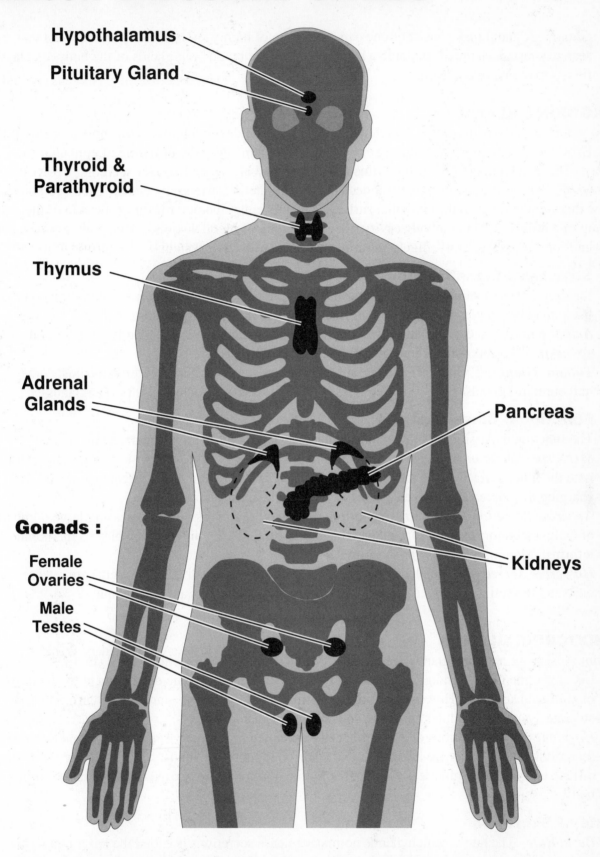

Hypothalamus

Pituitary Gland

Thyroid &
Parathyroid

Thymus

Adrenal
Glands

Pancreas

Gonads :

Female
Ovaries

Kidneys

Male
Testes

3

ENDOCRINE INTRODUCTION / Glands

Gland : A gland may consist of one cell or a group of highly specialized epithelial cells that secrete substances into ducts, onto a surface, or into the blood. All glands of the body are classified as exocrine or endocrine.

EXOCRINE GLANDS

Exo = outside. Exocrine glands secrete to the outside (outside the internal environment or ECF).

Exocrine glands are formed during embryonic development by the infolding of epithelial surfaces. This results in pockets or tubes lined with cells that are specialized for secreting a particular substance. These structures remain connected to the epithelial surfaces by ducts. Their secretions flow through the ducts to the epithelial surface, which is either the outer layer of the skin or the inner lining of a hollow organ or a body cavity (the inner lining of blood vessels, ducts, body cavities, and the interior of the respiratory, digestive, urinary, and reproductive systems).

Structural Classification

Structural classification is based on the shapes of the pockets : saccular or tubular. Each type of gland may be simple, branched, or compound; the tubular type may also be coiled.

Acinar Glands (saccular glands). Examples include : seminal vesicle glands (male reproductive system); oil-secreting sebaceous glands; and salivary glands.

Tubular Glands. Examples include : intestinal glands; gastric glands; uterine glands; bulbourethral glands (male reproductive system); and sudoriferous glands (sweat glands).

Functional Classification

The functional classification of exocrine glands is based on the secretion mechanism.

Merocrine Secretion Secretory products are released by exocytosis. A secretory vesicle fuses with the inner surface of the plasma membrane; the fused portion of the membrane opens, discharging the contents of the vesicle. Most exocrine glands are of this type.

Apocrine Secretion The entire top portion of a gland cell breaks away, releasing large numbers of Golgi (secretory) vesicles into the extracellular fluid (ECF); the ruptured plasma membrane reforms. Mammary glands are an example.

Holocrine Secretion The gland cell completely disintegrates; all of the contents are released at once and the cell is destroyed. Sebaceous (oil) glands of the skin are an example.

ENDOCRINE GLANDS

Endo = inside. Endocrine glands secrete their products into the extracellular fluid (ECF).

Like exocrine glands, endocrine glands are formed during embryonic development by the infolding of epithelial surfaces. However, during the formation of endocrine glands the connecting duct disintegrates, and the glandular epithelial cells become isolated clusters.

Hormones The secretions of endocrine cells are called hormones. Since there are no ducts, the secretions of these cells are released into the surrounding tissue fluids; from the tissue fluids they diffuse into nearby capillaries. Once in the blood, hormones are carried to all the tissues of the body.

Rate of Secretion

Basal Rate The rate at which glands normally release secretions is called the basal rate. This rate can be increased or decreased as the result of stimulation from nerves or hormones. The mechanism for altering the rate of secretion may involve the rate of synthesis or exocytosis.

GLANDS

Exocrine Glands

Exocrine gland cells secrete their products into ducts that empty at the skin surface or into the lumen of a hollow organ.

Acinar (Saccular) Glands

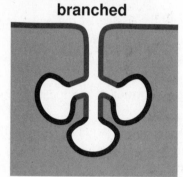

simple

seminal vesicle glands

branched

oil-secreting sebaceous glands

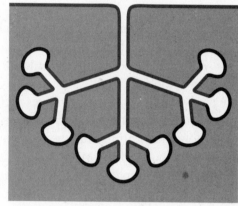

compound

salivary glands

Tubular Glands

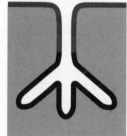

simple

intestinal glands

branched

gastric glands (stomach) uterine glands

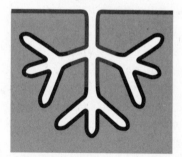

compound

bulbourethral glands (male reproductive system)

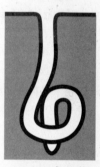

coiled

sweat glands (skin)

Endocrine Glands

Endocrine gland cells secrete hormones into nearby capillaries.

endocrine gland cells

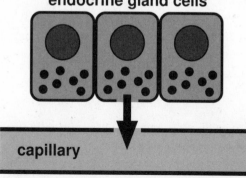

capillary

ENDOCRINE INTRODUCTION / Chemical Messengers

Chemical Messengers   Cells communicate with one another by means of chemicals; such chemicals are called chemical messengers.

HORMONES
Chemical messengers secreted by endocrine tissues are called hormones; they alter the physiological activity of specific target cells.

Target Cells   Hormones come into contact with all the tissues of the body, but they affect only specific cells. The cells affected by a particular hormone are referred to as the target cells of that hormone. They are recognized by the presence of hormone receptors on the outside of the plasma membrane or in the cytoplasm.

There are two main types of hormones : circulating hormones and local hormones.

Circulating Hormones (Endocrines)
Hormones that diffuse into the blood and act on *distant* target cells are called circulating hormones or endocrines.   Most circulating hormones are synthesized and secreted by specialized epithelial cells (endocrine cells) located in structures called endocrine glands. However, some endocrine cells are not found in structures limited to the production of hormones. For example, *enteroendocrine cells* are scattered among other epithelial cells that line the digestive tract; they secrete hormones involved in the digestive process.

Neurohormones   Hormones secreted by neurons are called neurohormones. Neurohormones are secreted by cells in the hypothalamus.

Local Hormones
Paracrines   Paracrines are chemical messengers that act on nearby cells. An example is histamine, which is released by mast cells and damaged tissue cells; it acts on nearby blood vessels, causing them to dilate.

Autocrines   Autocrines are chemical messengers that act on the same cells that secreted them. An example is interleukin-2 (IL-2).

> When a T cell (a type of white blood cell) is stimulated by the appropriate antigen and IL-1, it triggers the synthesis and secretion of IL-2 and also the synthesis of its own receptors for IL-2. Molecules of IL-2 are secreted by the T cells and bind to the surface receptors on the same T cells; this triggers mitosis, producing a clone of antigen-specific T cells.

SECOND MESSENGERS
Water-soluble hormones (peptides, proteins, and catecholamines) are unable to pass through plasma membranes, so a second messenger is needed to relay the message inside the cell.

cyclic AMP   The best known second messenger is cyclic AMP. The full name for cyclic AMP is *cyclic adenosine 3', 5' — monophosphate*; it is also known as *cAMP*. The binding of a hormone (first messenger) to a receptor on the outer surface of the plasma membrane activates an enzyme on the inner surface of the membrane that catalyzes the conversion of ATP into cAMP. The cAMP activates certain enzymes called *protein kinases*, which activate the proteins that mediate the cell's responses.

Other second messengers include calcium ions (Ca^{2+}), cyclic guanosine monophosphate (cGMP), inositol triphosphate (IP_3), and diacylglycerol (DAG).

NEUROTRANSMITTERS
Nerve cells communicate with each other and with effector cells (muscle cells and gland cells) by means of chemical messengers called neurotransmitters.

CHEMICAL MESSENGERS

Circulating Hormone

acts on distant target cells

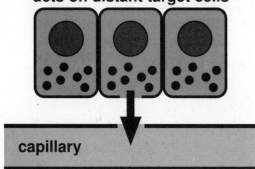

capillary

examples :
Aldosterone
Cortisol

Neurohormone

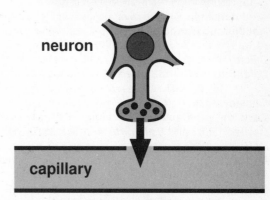

neuron

capillary

examples :
Antidiuretic Hormone
Gonadotropin-releasing Hormone

Autocrine

acts on the cell that secreted it

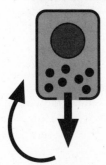

examples :
Interleukin-2
Tumor Necrosis Factor

Neurotransmitter

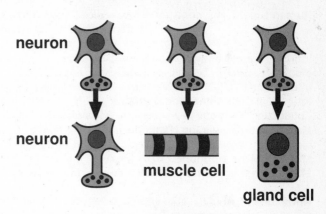

neuron

neuron

muscle cell

gland cell

examples :
Acetylcholine
Norepinephrine

Paracrine

acts on nearby cells

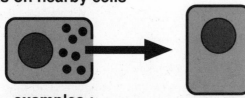

examples :
Histamine
Interferons

Adrenocorticotropic Hormone *(ACTH)* also called *Adrenocorticotropin* and *Corticotropin.*
Secreted by corticotrophs in the anterior pituitary gland.

Aldosterone Secreted by the adrenal cortex.

Angiotensin II Cleaved from Angiotensin I by enzymes located on capillary endothelial cells in the lungs.

Antidiuretic Hormone *(ADH)* also called *Vasopressin.* Secreted by the posterior pituitary.

Atrial Natriuretic Peptide *(ANP)* Secreted by cardiac muscle fibers of the atria (in the heart).

Calcitonin *(CT)* Secreted by parafollicular cells of the thyroid.

Calcitriol also called *1,25-dihydroxy cholecalciferol* or *1,25-dihydroxy vitamin* D_3.
Synthesized by a series of reactions that occur in the skin, liver, and kidneys.

Cholecystokinin *(CCK)* Secreted by enteroendocrine cells in the lining of the upper small intestine.

Corticotropin-Releasing Hormone *(CRH)* Secreted by neurons in the hypothalamus.

Cortisol also called *Hydrocortisone.* Secreted by cells of the zona fasciculata in the adrenal cortex.

Epinephrine also called *Adrenaline.* Secreted by chromaffin cells in the adrenal medulla.

Erythropoietin Secreted by cells in the kidneys and liver.

Estrogen Secreted by granulosa cells of maturing follicles in the ovaries.

Follicle-Stimulating Hormone *(FSH)* Secreted by gonadotrophs in the anterior pituitary.

Gastric Inhibitory Peptide *(GIP)* Secreted by enteroendocrine cells of the intestinal lining.

Gastrin Secreted by G-cells in the lining of the antrum of the stomach.

Glucagon Secreted by alpha cells in the pancreatic islets of the pancreas.

Gonadotropin-Releasing Hormone *(GnRH)* Secreted by neurons in the hypothalamus.

Growth Hormone-Inhibiting Hormone *(GHIH)* also called *Somatostatin.*
Secreted by neurons in the hypothalamus and D-cells in the pancreatic islets.

Growth Hormone-Releasing Hormone *(GHRH)* also called *Somatocrinin.*
Secreted by neurons in the hypothalamus.

Human Chorionic Gonadotropin *(hCG)* Secreted by the chorion of the placenta.

Human Chorionic Somatomammotropin *(hCS)* also called *Human Placental Lactogen (hPL).*
Secreted by the chorion of the placenta.

Human Growth Hormone *(hGH)* also called *Growth Hormone (GH)* and *Somatotropin.*
Secreted by somatotrophs in the anterior pituitary.

Inhibin Secreted by the testes, ovaries, and placenta.

Insulin Secreted by beta cells in the pancreatic islets.

Interleukin-1 *(IL-1)* Secreted by monocytes and macrophages.

Interstitial Cell-Stimulating Hormone *(ICSH)* Secreted by gonadotrophs in the anterior pituitary of males.

Luteinizing Hormone *(LH)* Secreted by gonadotrophs in the anterior pituitary of females.

Melanocyte-Stimulating Hormone *(MSH)* Secreted by corticotrophs in the anterior pituitary.

Melatonin Secreted by pinealocytes in the pineal gland.

MSH-Inhibiting Hormone *(MIH)* Secreted by neurons in the hypothalamus.

MSH-Releasing Hormone *(MRH)* Secreted by neurons in the hypothalamus.

Norepinephrine *(NE)* also called *Noradrenaline.* Secreted by chromaffin cells in the adrenal medulla.

Oxytocin *(OT)* Secreted by the posterior pituitary.

Pancreatic Polypeptide Secreted by F-cells in the pancreatic islets.

Parathyroid Hormone *(PTH)* also called *Parathormone.* Secreted by cells of the parathyroid glands.

Progesterone Secreted by follicle cells and luteal cells of the ovaries.

Prolactin *(PRL)* also called *Lactogenic Hormone.* Secreted by lactotrophs of the anterior pituitary.

Prolactin-Inhibiting Hormone *(PIH)* Secreted by neurons in the hypothalamus.

Prolactin-Releasing Hormone *(PRH)* Secreted by neurons in the hypothalamus.

Relaxin Secreted by cells of the corpus luteum in ovaries; and by cells in the placenta.

Secretin Secreted by enteroendocrine cells in the small intestine.

Somatomedins also called *insulinlike growth factors 1 and 2 (IGF-1 and IGF-2).* Secreted by the liver.

Testosterone Secreted by endocrinocytes (interstitial cells of Leydig) in the testes.

Thymosin Secreted by epithelial cells in the thymus.

Thyroid Hormones Includes two hormones : *Triiodothyronine* (T_3) and *Thyroxine* (T_4).
Secreted by follicle cells of the thyroid gland.

Thyroid-Stimulating Hormone *(TSH)* also called *Thyrotropin.* Secreted by thyrotrophs in the anterior pituitary.

Thyrotropin-Releasing Hormone *(TRH)* Secreted by neurons in the hypothalamus.

Tumor Necrosis Factor *(TNF)* Secreted by monocytes and macrophages.

HORMONE FUNCTIONS

Functions	Some Hormones Involved
Metabolic Rate	Thyroxine, Epinephrine, hGH, GHIH, Insulin, Glucagon
Digestion	Gastrin, Secretin, CCK, GHIH, Gastric Inhibitory Peptide
Reproduction	GnRH, FSH, LH, Prolactin, Progesterone, Estrogen, Inhibin, Oxytocin, Relaxin, Testosterone, Human Chorionic Gonadotropin, Human Chorionic Somatomammotropin
Blood Pressure	Epinephrine, Aldosterone, Antidiuretic Hormone, Angiotensin II, Histamine, Atrial Natriuretic Peptide
Calcium Balance	Calcitonin, Calcitriol, Parathyroid Hormone
Glucose Balance	Insulin, Glucagon, Epinephrine, GHIH
Salt & Water Balance	Aldosterone
Blood Cell Production	Erythropoietin (red blood cells), Thymosin (white blood cells)
Growth	Human Growth Hormone, Thyroid Hormones, Insulin, Testosterone, Estrogens
Immune Response	Interferons, Interleukins, Tumor Necrosis Factor, Lymphotoxin, Perforin, Thymosin
Stress Response	Cortisol, Epinephrine, Aldosterone, Antidiuretic Hormone, Growth Hormone, Glucagon

ENDOCRINE INTRODUCTION / Local Hormones

Local hormones act on nearby cells or on the same cells that secreted them. The following outline includes some examples of local hormones and their effects on target cells.

CYTOKINES
Cytokines are small protein hormones secreted by lymphocytes, monocytes, and macrophages.
The following are examples of cytokines that regulate immune responses.

Alpha and Beta Interferons *(Type I IFNs)*
Stimulate : T cell growth; activate NK cells (natural killer cells); production of antiviral enzymes in cells.

Gamma Interferon *(Type II IFN)*
Stimulates : phagocytosis by neutrophils and macrophages; production of antiviral enzymes in cells.

Interleukin-1 *(IL-1)*
Stimulates : T cell and B cell proliferation.

Interleukin-2 *(IL-2; T cell growth factor)*
Stimulates : cytotoxic T cell and B cell proliferation; activates NK cells (natural killer cells).

Interleukin-4 *(IL-4; B cell stimulating factor)*
Stimulates : B cells; growth of T cells; secretion of IgE antibodies from plasma cells.

Interleukin-5 *(IL-5)*
Stimulates : B cells; secretion of IgA antibodies from plasma cells.

Lymphotoxin *(LT)*
Action : kills cells by causing fragmentation of DNA.

Macrophage Migration Inhibiting Factor
Action : prevents macrophages from migrating away from the site of an infection.

Perforin
Action : perforates the cell membranes of target cells, killing them.

Transforming Growth Factor Beta *(TGF-beta)*
Action : inhibits the activation of T cells and macrophages.

Tumor Necrosis Factor *(TNF)*
Actions : stimulates the accumulation of leukocytes at the site of inflammation; activates leukocytes to kill microbes; stimulates macrophages to secrete IL-1.

GROWTH FACTORS
Local hormones that stimulate mitosis and/or differentiation are called growth factors.

Epidermal Growth Factor *(EGF)*
Stimulates : proliferation of epithelial cells, fibroblasts, neurons, and astrocytes.

Fibroblast Growth Factor *(FGF)*
Stimulates : proliferation of many types of cells derived from embryonic mesoderm.

Insulinlike Growth Factor *(IGF)*
Stimulates : growth of chondrocytes, fibroblasts, and other cells.

Nerve Growth Factor *(NGF)*
Stimulates : hypertrophy and differentiation of mature nerve cells.

Platelet-derived Growth Factor *(PDGF)*
Stimulates : proliferation of neuroglia, smooth muscle fibers, and fibroblasts.

Tumor Angiogenesis Factors *(TAFs)*
Stimulate : growth of new capillaries; organ regeneration; and wound healing.

HEMATOPOIETIC GROWTH FACTORS
Local hormones involved in blood cell formation (hematopoiesis) are called hematopoietic growth factors.

Granulocyte CSF *(G-CSF)*   *Stimulates* : development of neutrophils. (CSF = colony stimulating factor)

Granulocyte-Macrophage CSF *(GM-CSF)*   *Stimulates* : development of erythrocytes and leukocytes.

Interleukin-3 *(multi-CSF^a)*   *Stimulates* : pluripotent hematopoietic stem cells (hemocytoblasts).

Interleukin-5   *Stimulates* : development of eosinophils (type of white blood cell).

Interleukin-7   *Stimulates* : development of B cells (type of lymphocyte).

Macrophage CSF *(M-CSF)*   *Stimulates* : development of monocytes and macrophages.

Stem Cell Growth Factor *(steel factor)*   *Stimulates* : pluripotent hematopoietic stem cells (hemocytoblasts).

INTERFERONS

Virus-infected macrophages release interferons (IFNs). The interferons diffuse to neighboring cells and bind to surface receptors. This induces the uninfected cells to synthesize antiviral proteins that interfere with or inhibit viral replication.

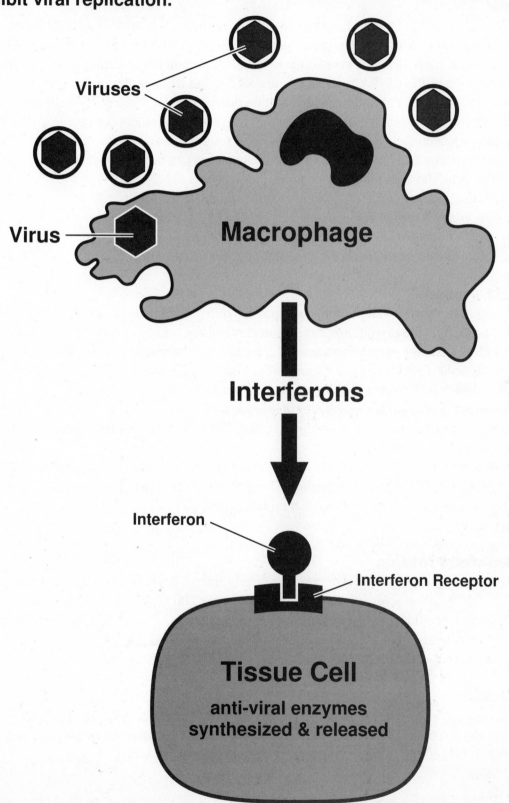

Viruses

Virus

Macrophage

Interferons

Interferon

Interferon Receptor

Tissue Cell

anti-viral enzymes
synthesized & released

ENDOCRINE INTRODUCTION / Chemistry of Hormones

There are four principal classes of hormones :
steroids; biogenic amines; peptides and proteins; and eicosanoids.

(1) Steroids

Steroids are a class of lipids; thus, they are fat-soluble and can pass through plasma membranes by diffusion. Being water-insoluble, they circulate in the blood bound to plasma proteins. All steroids have the same basic structure consisting of 4 linked carbon rings; variation in steroids is due to the composition of their side chains. They are all derived from cholesterol.

Steroids are synthesized by the adrenal cortex, the gonads, and the placenta. The adrenal cortex secretes glucocorticoids (95% of activity is due to cortisol) and mineralocorticoids (95% of activity is due to aldosterone). The ovaries secrete estrogens and progesterone, and the testes secrete testosterone. Calcitriol is produced by a series of reactions that start in the skin in response to stimulation by ultraviolet light; the final reactions occur in the liver and kidneys.

Glucocorticoids : mainly Cortisol (also cortisone and corticosterone).
Mineralocorticoids : mainly Aldosterone.
Sex Hormones : Estrogen, Progesterone, and Testosterone.
Calcitriol   (1,25-dihydroxy vitamin D_3 ; the active form of vitamin D).

(2) Biogenic Amines

Biogenic amines are small, water-soluble compounds derived from amino acids. Hormones of this chemical type include the thyroid hormones, catecholamines, and histamine (a local hormone). The thyroid hormones and the catecholamines are derived from the amino acid *tyrosine*. Histamine is derived from the amino acid *histidine*. Structurally, these are the simplest hormone molecules.

Thyroid Hormones : Triiodothyronine (T_3) and Thyroxine (T_4).
Catecholamines : Epinephrine and Norepinephrine (NE).
  Epinephrine (80% of secretions) Approximately 80% of the hormone produced by the adrenal medulla is epinephrine.
  Norepinephrine (20% of secretions) Some norepinephrine, which is epinephrine without a methyl group (— CH_3), is also secreted. The amounts of norepinephrine secreted are generally too small to exert significant actions on target cells.
Histamine.

(3) Peptides and Proteins

The great majority of all hormones are peptides or proteins. They range in size from very small peptides having only 3 amino acids to small proteins with over 200 amino acids. Most endocrinologists refer to all hormones that are peptides or proteins as "peptides." They include all of the hormones of the hypothalamus, pituitary gland, thyroid gland, parathyroid glands, stomach, small intestine, and pancreas. Growth factors belong to this chemical classification.

(4) Eicosanoids

Eicosanoids are derived from the 20-carbon fatty acid called arachidonic acid. They act primarily as local hormones (some are circulating hormones). They are synthesized by all cells of the body except red blood cells. The two major types of eicosanoids are :

Prostaglandins.
Leukotrienes.

HORMONE CLASSIFICATION : Steroids

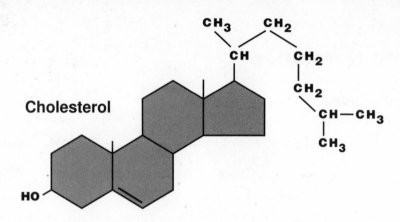

Cholesterol

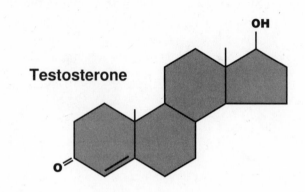

Testosterone

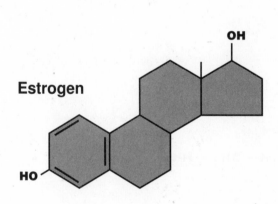

Estrogen

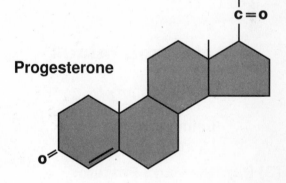

Progesterone

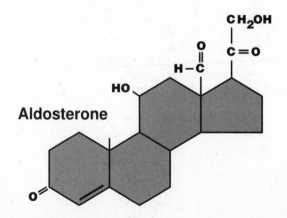

Aldosterone

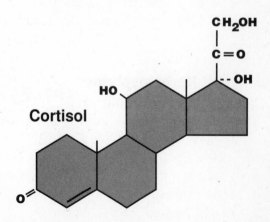

Cortisol

HORMONE CLASSIFICATION : Amines

Thyroid Hormones

Triiodothyronine
(T$_3$)

Thyroxine
(T$_4$)

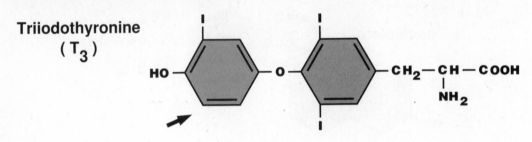

Catecholamines

Epinephrine
(Adrenaline)

Norepinephrine
(Noradrenaline)

HORMONE CLASSIFICATION : Peptides

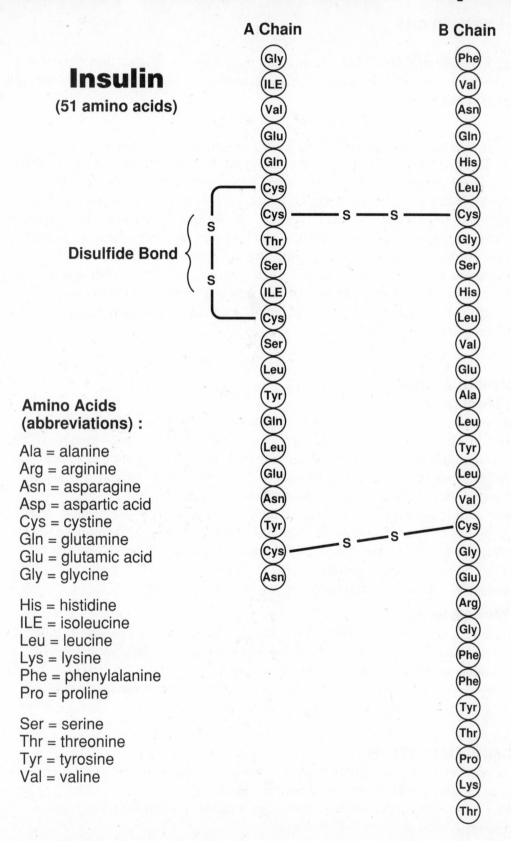

A Chain

B Chain

Insulin

(51 amino acids)

Disulfide Bond

**Amino Acids
(abbreviations) :**

Ala = alanine
Arg = arginine
Asn = asparagine
Asp = aspartic acid
Cys = cystine
Gln = glutamine
Glu = glutamic acid
Gly = glycine

His = histidine
ILE = isoleucine
Leu = leucine
Lys = lysine
Phe = phenylalanine
Pro = proline

Ser = serine
Thr = threonine
Tyr = tyrosine
Val = valine

ENDOCRINE INTRODUCTION / Hormone Receptors

LIGANDS and RECEPTORS

Ligands
A ligand is any ion or molecule that binds to a receptor protein by forces other than covalent bonds. All *chemical messengers* (circulating hormones, local hormones, second messengers, and neurotransmitters) are ligands.

Receptors
A receptor is a protein molecule that has a binding site for a chemical messenger.

Binding Sites   The binding site is a region of the protein that has a shape that is complementary to that of the chemical messenger, so that the chemical messenger can fit into the binding site. This property of a binding site is referred to as *chemical specificity*. The binding site also has charged and polarized regions that interact electrically with the ligand. The term *affinity* refers to how strongly a ligand is held to a binding site, based on how well the complementary shapes fit together and how strong the electrical forces of attraction are.

Target Cell Recognition   Some binding sites are specific for only one type of chemical messenger. This allows a chemical messenger to "identify" a particular protein receptor on the outer surface of a particular type of cell or in the cytoplasm of a particular type of cell. In this way a hormone can "recognize" its target cells.

RECEPTOR MODULATION

Allosteric Modulation
Some protein receptors have two binding sites : a regulatory site and a functional site.

Regulatory Site   If a ligand binds to a regulatory site, the distribution of forces within the receptor protein is altered, and, consequently, the shape of the second binding site (the functional site) is changed. A ligand that binds to a regulatory site is called a *modulator molecule*, because it modulates (changes) the shape and electrical nature of the functional site.

Functional Site   The functional site is responsible for the main function of the receptor. For example, if the protein receptor is an enzyme, the shape of the functional site determines whether the enyzme is activated or inactivated. The modulator molecule may increase or decrease the affinity of the functional site for its substrate.

(A substrate is a molecule that takes part in an enzyme-mediated reaction.)

Covalent Modulation
The shape of a protein receptor is also changed by phosphorylation. When a phosphate group is attached to a protein receptor by a covalent bond, the negative charge of the phosphate group alters the distribution of forces within the protein, changing its shape.

Protein Kinases   Protein kinases are enzymes that catalyze the transfer of phosphate from a molecule of ATP to a protein, changing the shape of the protein.

RECEPTOR CONCENTRATION
A target cell has between 2,000 and 100,000 receptors for a particular hormone. These receptors are constantly being synthesized and degraded (broken down).

Up-Regulation   An increase in the number of receptors is called up-regulation. The result is increased sensitivity of the target cell to the hormone.

Down-Regulation   A decrease in the number of receptors is called down-regulation. The result is decreased responsiveness of the target cell to the hormone.

RECEPTOR MODULATION

Allosteric Modulation

A modulator molecule binds to one binding site (the regulatory site) of a receptor; this alters the shape of a second binding site (the functional site).

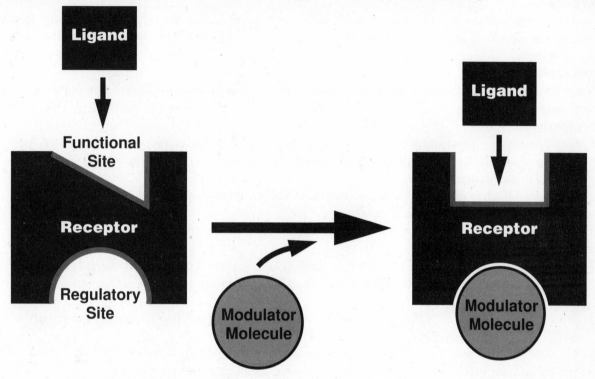

Covalent Modulation

A protein kinase catalyzes the binding of a phosphate group with a receptor; this alters the shape of the binding site.

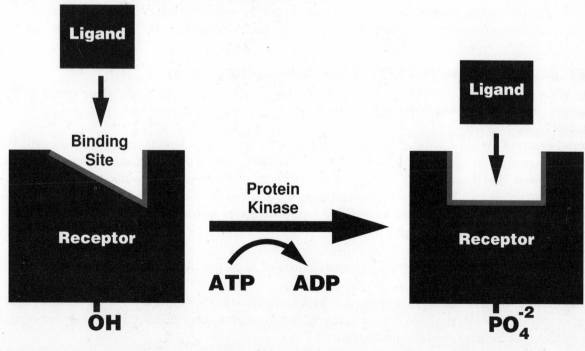

ENDOCRINE INTRODUCTION / Hormone Transport & Action

WATER-SOLUBLE HORMONES

Peptides and Proteins
Catecholamines (epinephrine and norepinephrine)

Transport

Because peptides, proteins, and catecholamines are polar molecules, they are soluble in the watery portion of blood plasma. They dissolve in the plasma and are transported to all regions of the body by the circulatory system.

Target Cell Action

Receptors : Receptors for water-soluble hormones are located on the outer surface of a cell's plasma membrane.

Mechanism :

(1) First Messenger The hormone is the first messenger; it combines with a receptor on the outer surface of the plasma membrane. Each receptor-hormone complex activates about 100 G-proteins located in the plasma membrane.

(2) G-Protein Each G-protein activates an enzyme called adenylate cyclase, which is located on the inner surface of the plasma membrane.

(3) Adenylate Cyclase Each adenylate cyclase catalyzes the conversion of about 1000 molecules of ATP to cyclic AMP.

(4) Second Messenger Cyclic AMP (cAMP) is the best known second messenger. Each cyclic AMP activates a type of enzyme called a protein kinase. The type of protein kinase activated varies with different target cells.

(5) Protein Kinase Each activated protein kinase initiates a series of reactions that alters the activity of a specific set of proteins (enzymes).

(6) Altered Cell Activities Each type of protein kinase regulates a particular cell activity, such as lipid breakdown, glycogen synthesis, protein synthesis, membrane transport, etc.

> *Amplification of Effects (approximate values) :*
> 1 hormone-receptor complex formed.
> 100 G-proteins activated (100 G-proteins by each hormone-receptor complex).
> 100 adenylate cyclases activated   (1 adenylate cyclase by each G-protein).
> 100,000 cyclic AMPs activated (1000 cAMPs formed by each adenylate cyclase).
> 100,000 protein kinases activated (1 protein kinase activated by each cAMP).
> 100,000,000 substrate molecules acted on (1000 molecules activated by each protein kinase).

WATER-INSOLUBLE HORMONES (Lipid-Soluble Hormones)

Steroids
Thyroid Hormones (triiodothyronine and thyroxine)

Transport

Bound Fraction When water-insoluble hormones enter the blood, they bind to plasma proteins called *transport proteins*; the new hormone-protein complex is soluble in the watery portion of blood.

Free Fraction The 0.1 to 10% of the lipid-soluble hormone that does not bind to transport proteins is called the free fraction. These free hormones diffuse out of capillaries and interact with target cell receptors. An equilibrium exists between the free and bound hormones: as free hormones bind to receptors, transport proteins release additional hormones.

Target Cell Action

Receptors : The receptors for steroid hormones are located in the cytoplasm of the target cells (in the cytosol or nucleoplasm).

Mechanism : Because steroids are lipids, they pass easily through the bilipid layer of the plasma membranes and bind to their receptors. The receptor-hormone complex alters the activity of genes that regulate the synthesis of particular proteins (enzymes).

HORMONE ACTION

Some peptide hormones act via cyclic AMP to increase or decrease enzyme activity.

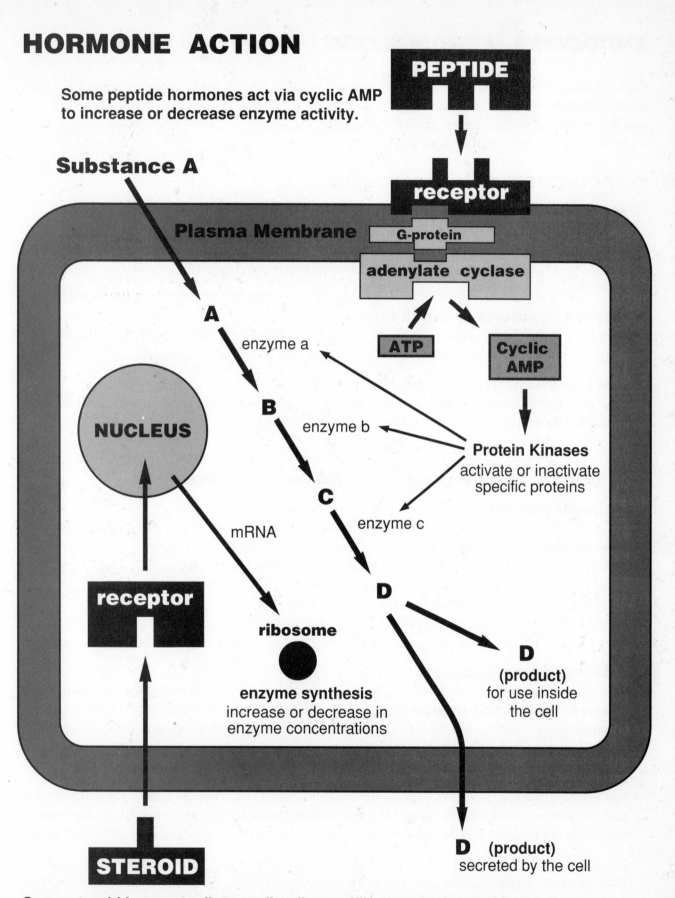

Substance A

PEPTIDE

receptor

Plasma Membrane

G-protein

adenylate cyclase

A

enzyme a

ATP

Cyclic AMP

NUCLEUS

B

enzyme b

Protein Kinases
activate or inactivate
specific proteins

C

enzyme c

mRNA

D

receptor

ribosome

D
(product)
for use inside
the cell

enzyme synthesis
increase or decrease in
enzyme concentrations

STEROID

D (product)
secreted by the cell

Some steroid hormones "turn on" or "turn off" genes in the nucleus,
causing an increase or decrease in the synthesis of specific proteins (enzymes).

ENDOCRINE INTRODUCTION / Target Cell Responses

The initial step leading to a target cell's ultimate responses to a hormone is called *receptor activation*; it is the binding of a hormone to its receptor protein in the target cell. The ultimate target cell responses are due to changes in the shape (and therefore the activity) of particular cell proteins or to changes in the concentration of particular proteins.

TYPES OF TARGET CELL RESPONSES

Membrane Transport
A change in the permeability of a plasma membrane to a particular ion results from the altered shape of the proteins that form the walls of the ion channels. A change in the rate of active transport or facilitated transport through a plasma membrane results from the altered shape of the proteins involved in the transport mechanism.

Rate of Synthesis or Breakdown
A change in the rate of synthesis or breakdown of a particular substance results from the altered shape or concentration of proteins (enzymes) in the relevant metabolic pathway.

Rate or Strength of Muscle Contraction
A change in the rate or strength of muscle contractions in smooth or cardiac muscle cells results from the altered shape of contractile proteins in the muscle.

AN EXAMPLE : Cardiac Muscle Cell Response to Epinephrine

Sequence of Events
Epinephrine binds to beta-adrenergic receptors in the plasma membrane of myocardial cells.
The activated receptor interacts with a G-protein in the plasma membrane.
The G-protein activates membrane-bound adenylate cyclase (an enzyme).
Adenylate cyclase catalyzes the conversion of ATP into cyclic AMP in the cytosol.
Cyclic AMP activates *cAMP-dependent protein kinase*.
Activated protein kinase phosphorylates at least three different proteins.
As a result of phosphorylation (adding a phosphate group), the protein activities are altered.

Altered Cell Proteins
(1) Calcium Ion Channels   Plasma membrane proteins that control slow calcium channels are activated. As a result, a greater number of slow calcium channels open during excitation; more calcium ions enter the cell and bind to troponin, which results in an increase in the number of actin-myosin cross-bridge attachments. The ultimate effect is a more forceful contraction.

(2) Sarcoplasmic Reticulum   Plasma-bound proteins that control an *ATP-dependent calcium-uptake pump* are activated. As a result, the active transport of calcium is stimulated and more calcium ions are pumped into the sarcoplasmic reticulum for storage. Consequently, more calcium ions are released into the cytosol during excitation, resulting in a more forceful contraction.

(3) Myosin   The contractile proteins that form the thick filaments in muscle fibers are altered. This causes an increase in the rate at which cross-bridges cycle. The ultimate effect is an increase in the velocity of contraction.

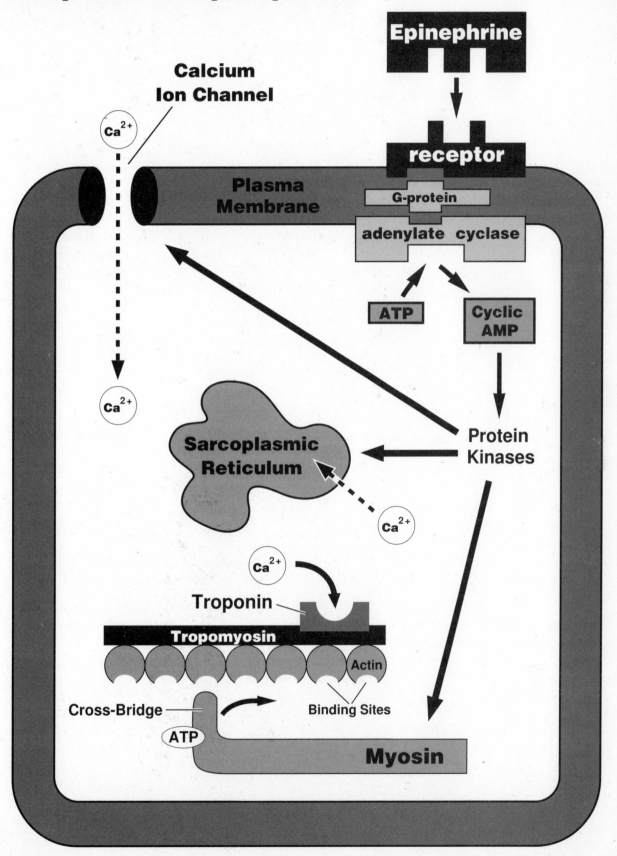

2 Endocrine Tissues

Hypothalamus *24*
1. Tropic Hormones   releasing hormones : GHRH, PRH, GnRH, TRH, CRH, and MRH
                                       inhibiting hormones : GHIH, PIH, and MIH
2. Hormones released by the Posterior Pituitary Gland : ADH and OT

Pituitary Gland *26*
1. Pituitary Gland Structures : basic structures and cell types
2. Posterior Pituitary Gland : Antidiuretic Hormone (ADH) and Oxytocin (OT)

Anterior Pituitary Gland *28*
1. Human Growth Hormone (hGH)
2. Prolactin (PRL)
3. Follicle-Stimulating Hormone (FSH)
4. Luteinizing Hormone (LH)
5. Thyroid-Stimulating Hormone (TSH)
6. Adrenocorticotropic Hormone (ACTH)
7. Melanocyte-Stimulating Hormone (MSH)

Adrenal Glands *30*
1. Adrenal Cortex : Cortisol, Aldosterone, and Sex Hormones
2. Adrenal Medulla : Epinephrine and Norepinephrine (NE)

Thyroid and Parathyroid Glands *32*
1. Thyroid Gland : Thyroid Hormones (TH) and Calcitonin (CT)
2. Parathyroid Gland : Parathyroid Hormone (PTH)

Stomach and Small Intestine *34*
1. Stomach : Gastrin
2. Small Intestine : Cholecystokinin (CCK), Secretin, and Gastric Inhibitory Peptide (GIP)

Pancreatic Islets *36*
1. Glucagon   2. Insulin   3. GHIH   4. Pancreatic Polypeptide

Kidneys *38*
1. Erythropoietin   2. Calcitriol   3. Angiotensin II

Testes *40*
1. Testosterone   2. Inhibin

Ovaries and Placenta *42*
1. Ovaries : Estrogens, Progesterone, Inhibin, and Relaxin
2. Placenta : Estrogens, Progesterone, Inhibin, Relaxin, hCG, and hCS

Pineal Gland, Heart, and Liver *44*
1. Pineal Gland : Melatonin
2. Heart : Atrial Natriuretic Factor
3. Liver : Somatomedins (IGF-1 and IGF-2)

Thymus Gland, Lymphocytes, Macrophages, and Monocytes *46*
1. Thymus : Thymosin, Thymic Humoral Factor, Thymic Factor, and Thymopoietin
2. Lymphocytes : Gamma Interferon and Interleukin-2
3. Macrophages and Monocytes : Tumor Necrosis Factor and Interleukin-1

ENDOCRINE TISSUES / Hypothalamus

TROPIC HORMONES

Neurons in the hypothalamus secrete *tropic hormones* — hormones that stimulate or inhibit the release of hormones from their target cells. In the hypothalamus the tropic hormones are secreted into capillary beds and carried by the *hypophyseal portal veins* to their target cells in the anterior pituitary (adenohypophysis).

Releasing Hormones

(1) GHRH (Growth Hormone-Releasing Hormone) also called *Somatocrinin*.
target cells : somatotrophs in the anterior pituitary.
action : stimulates the release of human growth hormone (hGH / GH / somatotropin).

(2) PRH (Prolactin-Releasing Hormone)
target cells : lactotrophs in the anterior pituitary.
action : stimulates the release of prolactin (PRL).

(3) GnRH (Gonadotropin-Releasing Hormone)
target cells : gonadotrophs in the anterior pituitary.
action : stimulates the release of follicle-stimulating (FSH) and luteinizing hormone (LH).

(4) TRH (Thyrotropin-Releasing Hormone)
target cells : thyrotrophs in the anterior pituitary.
action : stimulates the release of thyroid-stimulating hormone (TSH).

(5) CRH (Corticotropin-Releasing Hormone)
target cells : corticotrophs in the anterior pituitary.
action : stimulates the release of adrenocorticotropic hormone (ACTH).

(6) MRH (Melanocyte-Stimulating Hormone Releasing Hormone)
target cells : corticotrophs in the anterior pituitary.
action : stimulates the release of melanocyte-stimulating hormone (MSH).

Inhibiting Hormones

(1) GHIH (Growth Hormone-Inhibiting Hormone) also called *Somatostatin*.
target cells : somatotrophs in the anterior pituitary.
action : inhibits the release of human growth hormone (hGH / GH / somatotropin).

(2) PIH (Prolactin-Inhibiting Hormone)
target cells : lactotrophs in the anterior pituitary.
action : inhibits the release of prolactin (PRL).

(3) MIH (Melanocyte-Stimulating Hormone Inhibiting Hormone)
target cells : corticotrophs in the anterior pituitary.
action : inhibits the release of melanocyte-stimulating hormone (MSH).

HORMONES RELEASED BY THE POSTERIOR PITUITARY GLAND

ADH (Antidiuretic Hormone, also called Vasopressin) and **OT** (Oxytocin)

Neuron cell bodies located in the supraoptic and paraventricular nuclei of the hypothalamus have long axons that extend to the posterior pituitary gland, where antidiuretic hormone and oxytocin are released from their axon terminals into the bloodstream.

HYPOTHALAMUS

Neurons in the hypothalamus secrete neurohormones.

9 tropic hormones travel to the anterior pituitary gland via portal vessels.
ADH and oxytocin travel down long axons
and are released into the general circulation in the posterior pituitary.

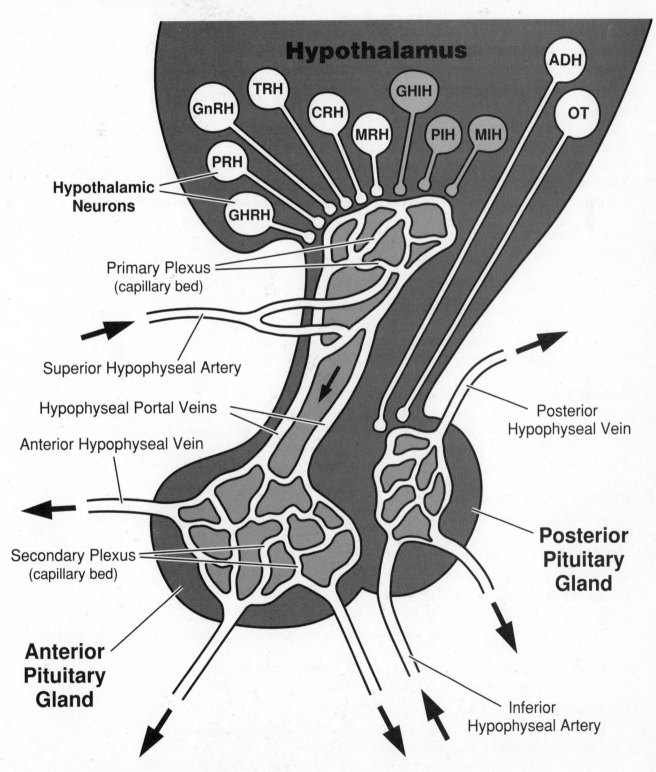

25

ENDOCRINE TISSUES / Pituitary Gland

PITUITARY GLAND STRUCTURES

Basic Structures (alphabetical order)

Adenohypophysis (*adeno* = glandular) : the anterior pituitary gland (anterior lobe).

Anterior Hypophyseal Veins : carry blood and hormones from the secondary plexus toward target cells.

Hypophyseal Portal Veins : vessels that carry blood from the primary plexus to the secondary plexus.

Hypophysis : another name for the pituitary gland.

Inferior Hypophyseal Arteries: vessels that supply the posterior pituitary.

Infundibulum : a stalklike structure that connects the pituitary to the hypothalamus.

Median Eminence : the region at the base of the hypothalamus from which portal vessels arise.

Neurohypophysis (*neuro* = nervous) : the posterior pituitary gland (posterior lobe).

Pars Intermedia : a nonvascular region between the anterior and posterior lobes.

Posterior Hypophyseal Veins : carry blood and hormones from the posterior pituitary toward target cells.

Primary Plexus : a network of capillaries in the median eminence.

Secondary Plexus : a network of capillaries in the anterior pituitary formed by hypophyseal portal veins.

Sella Turcica (*Turk's saddle*) :   a depression in the sphenoid bone that houses the pituitary gland.

Superior Hypophyseal Arteries : vessels that carry blood into the base of the hypothalamus.

Cell Types

Anterior Lobe

   (1) Somatotrophs : secrete Human Growth Hormone (hGH).

   (2) Lactotrophs : secrete Prolactin (PRL).

   (3) Corticotrophs : secrete Adrenocorticotropic Hormone (ACTH);
                      secrete Melanocyte-Stimulating Hormone (MSH).

   (4) Thyrotrophs : secrete Thyroid-Stimulating Hormone (TSH).

   (5) Gonadotrophs : secrete Follicle-Stimulating Hormone (FSH).
                      secrete Luteinizing Hormone (LH).

Posterior Lobe

   (1) Pituicytes : supporting cells that resemble neuroglia; associated with the neurosecretory cells.

   (2) Axon Terminals of Neurosecretory Cells : The posterior lobe of the pituitary gland contains
        about 5000 axon terminals that store and secrete hormones; the neuron cell bodies are
        located in the supraoptic and paraventricular nuclei of the the hypothalamus.

POSTERIOR PITUITARY GLAND

   Neuron cell bodies located in the supraoptic and paraventricular nuclei of the hypothalamus have long
axons that extend to the posterior pituitary where antidiuretic hormone (ADH /vasopressin) and oxytocin (OT)
are released from their axon terminals into the bloodstream. These hormones are *synthesized* in the hypothalamus and *secreted* by the posterior pituitary.

   (1) Antidiuretic Hormone (ADH; also called *vasopressin*)   secreted by neuron axon terminals
      secretion stimulated by : low water concentration of blood (dehydration), pain, stress, trauma,
         anxiety, nicotine, morphine, some anesthetics, tranquilizers, acetylcholine (neurotransmitter).
         (Secretion of ADH is inhibited by alcohol.)
      *actions : increases water reabsorption by the kidneys (raises blood pressure);
         causes constriction of arterioles during severe hemorrhage.*

   (2) Oxytocin (OT)   secreted by neuron axon terminals
      secretion stimulated by : uterine distension; stimulation of nipples (suckling).
      *actions : stimulates uterine contractions during labor;
         stimulates milk ejection (contraction of myoepithelial cells in mammary glands).*

PITUITARY GLAND

Location

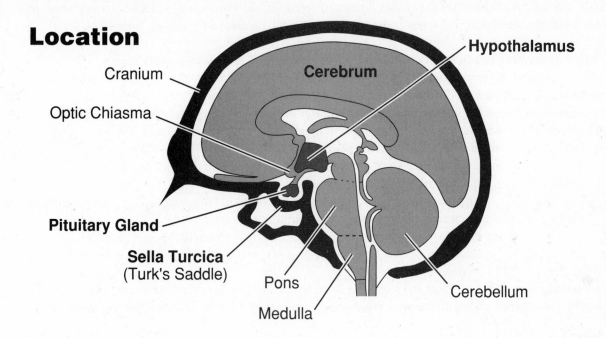

Cranium

Optic Chiasma

Pituitary Gland

Sella Turcica
(Turk's Saddle)

Cerebrum

Hypothalamus

Pons

Medulla

Cerebellum

Posterior Pituitary Gland

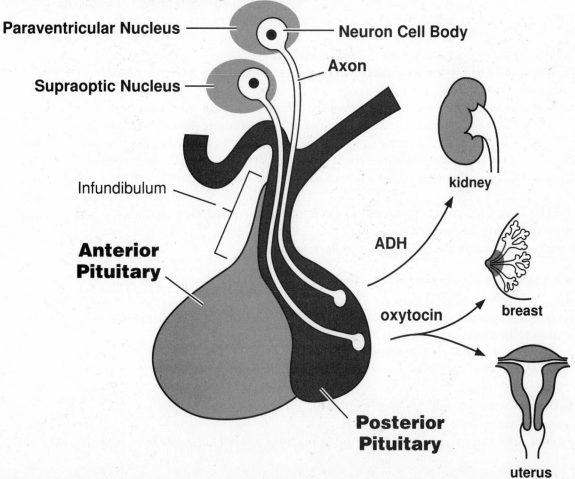

Paraventricular Nucleus

Supraoptic Nucleus

Infundibulum

**Anterior
Pituitary**

Neuron Cell Body

Axon

kidney

ADH

oxytocin

breast

**Posterior
Pituitary**

uterus

ENDOCRINE TISSUES / Anterior Pituitary Gland

The anterior lobe of the pituitary gland consists largely of epithelial cells arranged in blocks around many thin-walled blood vessels. Five principal types of anterior pituitary cells secrete seven major hormones.

(1) hGH (Human Growth Hormone or *Growth Hormone/GH or Somatotropin*)
        secreted by somatotrophs
secretion controlled by : GHRH, GHIH, and TRH.
actions : increases blood glucose levels; stimulates protein synthesis and growth of body cells.
   body cells : increases the rate of amino acid uptake and protein synthesis;
                increases the use of amino acids and fatty acids for ATP synthesis;
                decreases the uptake of glucose and its utilization for ATP synthesis.
   bone : stimulates protein synthesis (bone growth).
   adipose tissue : stimulates the breakdown of triglycerides into fatty acids and glycerol (lipolysis).
   liver : stimulates secretion of somatomedins (insulinlike growth factor / IGF);
                increases the rate of conversion of glycogen and noncarbohydrates into glucose.

(2) PRL (Prolactin)   secreted by lactotrophs
secretion controlled by : PRH and PIH (regulated by the sucking action of the infant).
action : initiates and maintains milk synthesis and secretion into the alveoli of mammary glands.

(3) FSH (Follicle-Stimulating Hormone)   secreted by gonadotrophs
secretion controlled by : GnRH.
actions : regulates gamete production and sex hormone secretion.
   female ovaries : initiates the development of ova (eggs) and the secretion of estrogens.
   male testes : stimulates spermatogenesis (production of sperm).

(4) LH (Luteinizing Hormone)   secreted by gonadotrophs
In males luteinizing hormone is called *interstitial cell-stimulating hormone (ICSH)*.
secretion controlled by : GnRH.
actions : stimulates the secretion of estrogens, progesterone, and testosterone.
   female ovaries : stimulates the secretion of estrogens (during the follicular phase);
                the LH surge triggers ovulation (about the 14th day of the menstrual cycle);
                stimulates the secretion of progesterone (during the luteal phase).
   male testes : stimulates the secretion of testosterone by the interstitial cells of Leydig.

(5) TSH (Thyroid-Stimulating Hormone or *Thyrotropin*)   secreted by thyrotrophs
secretion controlled by : TRH.
actions : stimulates secretion of thyroid hormones.

(6) ACTH (Adrenocorticotropic Hormone or *Corticotropin* or *Adrenocorticotropin*)
        secreted by corticotrophs
secretion controlled by : CRH, ADH, Epinephrine, Interleukin-1, and Lymphokines.
actions : stimulates the release of cortisol and aldosterone.
   zona fasciculata : stimulates the secretion of cortisol.
   zona glomerulosa : stimulates the secretion of aldosterone.

(7) MSH (Melanocyte-Stimulating Hormone)   secreted by corticotrophs
secretion controlled by : MRH and MIH.
action : stimulates dispersion of melanin granules in amphibians; role in humans is unknown.

ANTERIOR PITUITARY GLAND

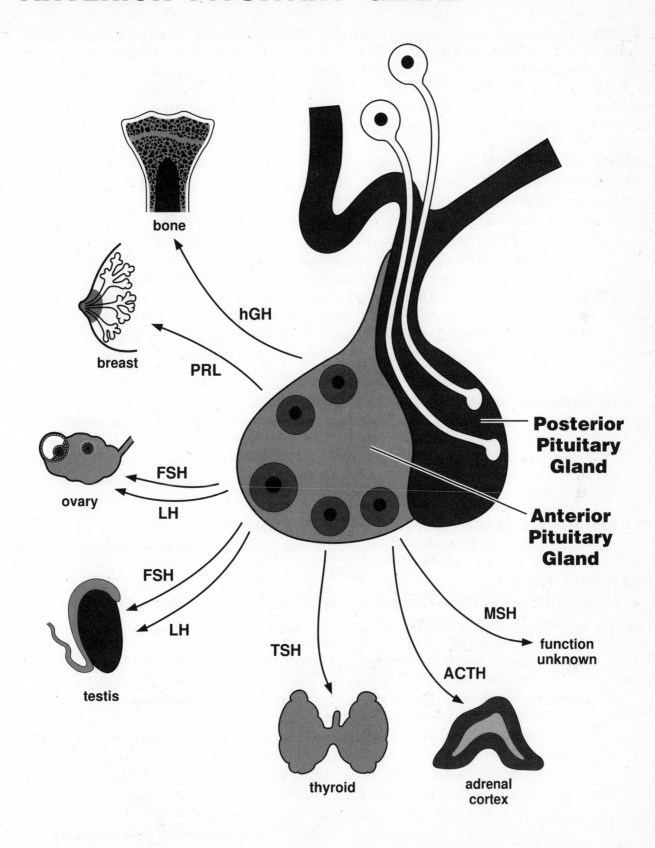

bone

breast

hGH

PRL

ovary

FSH

LH

FSH

LH

testis

TSH

thyroid

ACTH

adrenal
cortex

MSH

function
unknown

**Posterior
Pituitary
Gland**

**Anterior
Pituitary
Gland**

ENDOCRINE TISSUES / Adrenal Glands

There are two adrenal glands, one above each kidney. The outer portion of each gland is called the adrenal cortex; the inner portion is called the adrenal medulla. Each gland is surrounded by a capsule. The adrenal cortex has three layers: the outer layer is called the zona glomerulosa and secretes *mineralocorticoids* (mainly aldosterone); the middle layer is called the zona fasciculata and secretes *glucocorticoids* (mainly cortisol); the inner layer is called the zona reticularis and secretes *gonadocorticoids* (sex hormones). The adrenal medulla is in the center of the adrenal gland; it secretes epinephrine (80%) and norepinephrine (20%).

ADRENAL CORTEX
Cortisol   also called *Hydrocortisone.*   secreted by cells in the zona fasciculata
secretion stimulated by : ACTH.
actions : increases plasma glucose, fatty acid, and amino acid levels;
responds to stress; counters the inflammatory response.
   body cells : inhibits glucose uptake (but not by brain cells).
   skeletal muscle : conversion of proteins into amino acids (protein catabolism).
   adipose tissue : conversion of triglycerides into fatty acids and glycerol (lipolysis).
   liver : conversion of amino acids into glucose (gluconeogenesis).
   lymphocytes : inhibits the inflammatory response and antibody production.
   connective tissue : retards regeneration; slows wound healing.
   arterioles : increases vasoconstriction in response to epinephrine.

Aldosterone   secreted by cells in the zona glomerulosa
secretion stimulated by : ACTH; decreased plasma sodium; increased plasma potassium;
                              angiotensin II (renin-angiotensin pathway).
actions : increases plasma sodium (and water) levels; decreases plasma potassium levels.
   kidneys :   increases reabsorption of sodium (decreases excretion of sodium);
                increases secretion of potassium (increases excretion of potassium).

Sex Hormones   secreted by cells in the zona reticularis
The adrenal cortex secretes small amounts of sex hormones (estrogens and androgens).

ADRENAL MEDULLA
Epinephrine and Norepinephrine (NE)   also called *Adrenaline* and *Noradrenaline.*
      secreted by chromaffin cells
secretion stimulated by : preganglionic sympathetic nerves.
actions : mimics the effects caused by the sympathetic division of the ANS;
increases blood concentrations of glucose, fatty acids, and glycerol.
   body cells : increases the rate of metabolism (heat produced by the calorigenic effect).
   skeletal muscle : decreases glucose uptake; increases efficiency of contractions.
   adipose tissue : conversion of triglycerides into fatty acids and glycerol (lipolysis).
   liver : conversion of glycogen and noncarbohydrates into glucose.
   heart : increases heart rate and force of contractions (increases blood pressure).
   lungs : bronchioles dilate (increases oxygen intake by lungs); stimulates ventilation.
   eyes : stimulates contraction of radial muscles in the iris (pupils dilate).
   anterior pituitary : stimulates release of ACTH (increases cortisol and aldosterone).
   blood plasma : blood clots more quickly.
   arterioles : vasoconstriction of vessels to most tissues; vasodilation of vessels to muscles.

ADRENAL GLANDS

Adrenal Cortex : zona fasciculata secretes cortisol
zona glomerulosa secretes aldosterone
zona reticularis secretes sex hormones

Adrenal Medulla : secretes epinephrine and norepinephrine

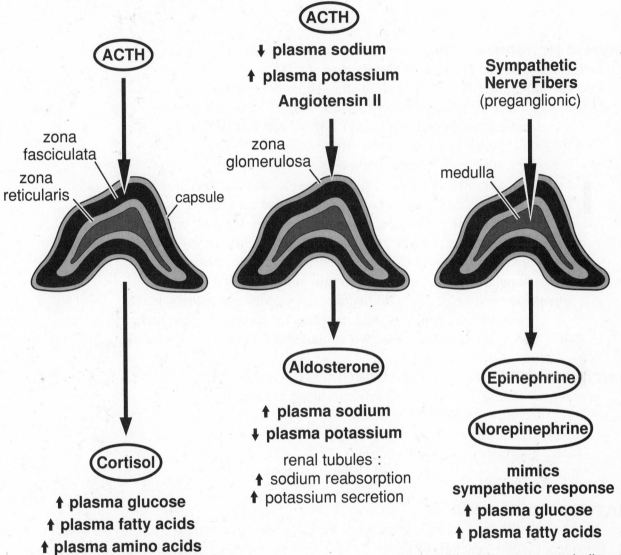

↑ **plasma glucose**
↑ **plasma fatty acids**
↑ **plasma amino acids**
↓ **inflammatory response**

body cells : inhibits glucose uptake
skeletal muscle : proteins to amino acids
adipose tissue : triglycerides to fatty acids
liver : amino acids to glucose
lymphocytes : inhibits antibody production
connective tissue : retards regeneration
arterioles : vasoconstriction
            (in response to epinephrine)

↑ **plasma sodium**
↓ **plasma potassium**
renal tubules :
↑ sodium reabsorption
↑ potassium secretion

mimics
sympathetic response
↑ **plasma glucose**
↑ **plasma fatty acids**

body cells : increases matabolic rate
skeletal muscle : decreases glucose uptake
adipose tissue : triglycerides to fatty acids
liver : glycogen to glucose
heart : increases cardiac output
lungs : bronchioles dilate
eyes : pupils dilate
anterior pituitary : stimulates ACTH release
blood plasma : blood clots more quickly
arterioles : vasoconstriction
            (except in skeletal muscle)

ENDOCRINE TISSUES / Thyroid and Parathyroid Glands

THYROID GLAND

The thyroid gland, located in the neck, actually secretes 3 different hormones. Two of them are collectively known as thyroid hormones (TH): triiodothyronine (T_3) and thyroxine (T_4). The subscripts in the abbreviations indicate the number of iodine atoms in the molecule. Thyroxine has one more iodine atom than triiodothyronine; otherwise they are identical molecules. The third hormone produced by the thyroid gland is calcitonin.

Thyroid Hormones (TH)   secreted by follicular cells
Triiodothyronine (T_3) and Thyroxine (T_4)
secretion stimulated by : TSH (thyroid-stimulating hormone).
actions : increase metabolic rate and cardiac output; stimulate growth;
        development, growth, and activity of the nervous system.
  body cells : increases the metabolic rate (calorigenic effect);
        stimulates protein synthesis;
        stimulates growth (facilitates the effects of human growth hormone);
        stimulates synthesis of the enyzme that runs the Na^+/K^+ pump;
        stimulates the use of glucose and oxygen for ATP production.
  adipose tissue : conversion of triglycerides to fatty acids and glycerol (lipolysis).
  heart : increases cardiac output (increases heart rate and stroke volume).
  brain : stimulates development of the brain in the fetus and infant.
  sympathetic nervous system : facilitates activity of the sympathetic nerves.
        (stimulates synthesis of beta receptors for epinephrine and norepinephrine).
  gallbladder : stimulates the secretion of cholesterol in the bile (lowers plasma levels).

Calcitonin (CT)   secreted by parafollicular cells (C cells)
secretion stimulated by : increased levels of blood calcium.
actions : decreases blood calcium levels.
  bone : increases the rate of calcium deposited in bone.
  kidneys : increases calcium excretion.

PARATHYROID GLANDS

There are two parathyroid glands embedded in the posterior portion of each lobe of the thyroid gland. Each parathyroid gland has two distinct cell types : the principal cells (also called chief cells), which secrete PTH, and the oxyphil cells (function unknown).

Parathyroid Hormone (PTH)   also called *Parathormone*.
  secreted by principal cells
secretion stimulated by : decreased levels of blood calcium.
actions : increases blood calcium levels; decreases blood phosphate levels.
  bone : increases the rate of calcium release from bones (stimulates osteoclasts).
  kidneys : increases calcium reabsorption (from urine into the blood);
        increases phosphate excretion in the urine;
        promotes the formation of calcitriol (active form of vitamin D).
  small intestine : increases dietary calcium and magnesium absorption.

THYROID and PARATHYROID GLANDS

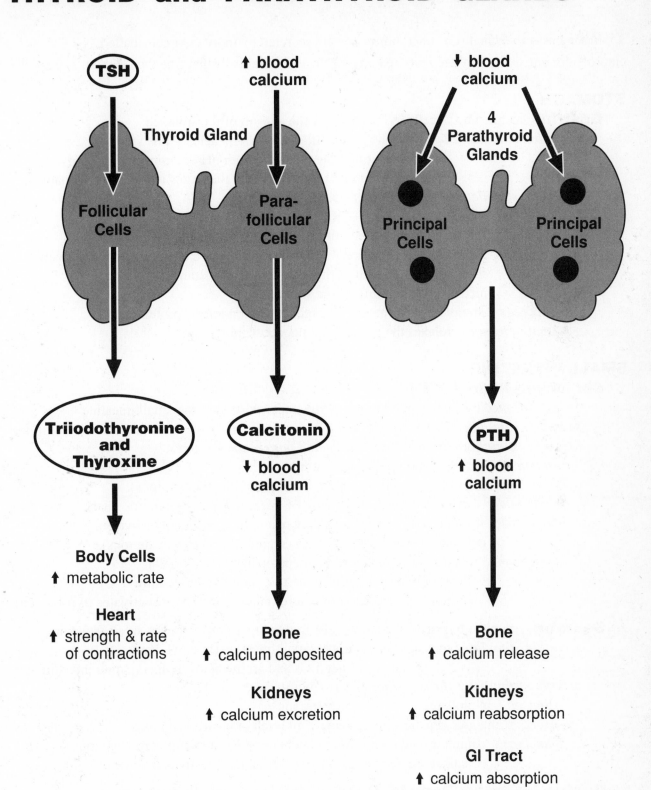

TSH

↑ blood calcium

↓ blood calcium

Thyroid Gland

4 Parathyroid Glands

Follicular Cells

Para-follicular Cells

Principal Cells

Principal Cells

Triiodothyronine and Thyroxine

Calcitonin
↓ blood calcium

PTH
↑ blood calcium

Body Cells
↑ metabolic rate

Heart
↑ strength & rate of contractions

Bone
↑ calcium deposited

Kidneys
↑ calcium excretion

Bone
↑ calcium release

Kidneys
↑ calcium reabsorption

GI Tract
↑ calcium absorption

ENDOCRINE TISSUES / Stomach and Small Intestine

In the gastrointestinal (GI) tract, hormones are secreted by individual cells called enteroendocrine cells; they are scattered among the epithelial cells that line the GI tract.

STOMACH
Gastrin   secreted by G-cells in the lining of the antrum of the stomach

secretion stimulated by : presence of peptides and amino acids in the stomach; distension of the stomach; high pH of stomach contents; increased rate of discharge by the vagus nerve (parasympathetic).

actions : stimulates the secretion of gastric juice.

esophagus : causes contraction of the lower esophageal sphincter.

stomach : stimulates the secretion of HCl from parietal cells; stimulates the secretion of pepsinogen (inactive enzyme) from chief cells; stimulates the growth of the gastric mucosa (stomach lining); increases the motility of the stomach.

pancreas : stimulates insulin and glucagon secretion after a protein meal.

small intestine : relaxes the pyloric and ileocecal sphincters.

SMALL INTESTINE
Cholecystokinin (CCK)

secreted by I-cells in the lining of the upper portion of the small intestine

secretion stimulated by : the presence of amino acids and fatty acids in the small intestine.

actions : stimulates the secretion of bile and pancreatic enzymes.

stomach : inhibits gastric peristalsis (motility).

liver : enhances the action of secretin (secretion of bicarbonate ions).

gallbladder : causes contraction (release of bile into the common bile duct).

pancreas : stimulates the secretion of pancreatic juice rich in digestive enzymes; enhances the action of secretin (secretion of bicarbonate ions).

duodenum : relaxes the sphincter of the hepatopancreatic ampulla, allowing bile to flow from the liver into the duodenum; increases the secretion of enterokinase (enzyme that activates trypsinogen).

Secretin   secreted by enteroendocrine cells in the upper portion of the small intestine

secretion stimulated by : acid in the upper small intestine (low pH due to HCl) presence of peptides and amino acids in upper small intestine.

actions : stimulates the secretion of bicarbonate ions.

stomach : inhibits the secretion of gastric juice.

liver : stimulates hepatic cells to secrete bile rich in bicarbonate ions.

pancreas : stimulates the secretion of pancreatic juice rich in bicarbonate ions; enhances the action of CCK (secretion of digestive enzymes).

Gastric Inhibitory Peptide (GIP)   secreted by enteroendocrine cells

secretion stimulated by : glucose and fat in the duodenum.

actions : inhibits the secretion of gastric juices.

stomach : inhibits secretion of gastric juices and gastric peristalsis (motility).

pancreas : stimulates insulin secretion.

STOMACH and SMALL INTESTINE

Enteroendocrine cells in the lining of the digestive tract secrete hormones. Hepatic cells and cells lining the pancreatic ducts secrete bicarbonate ions.

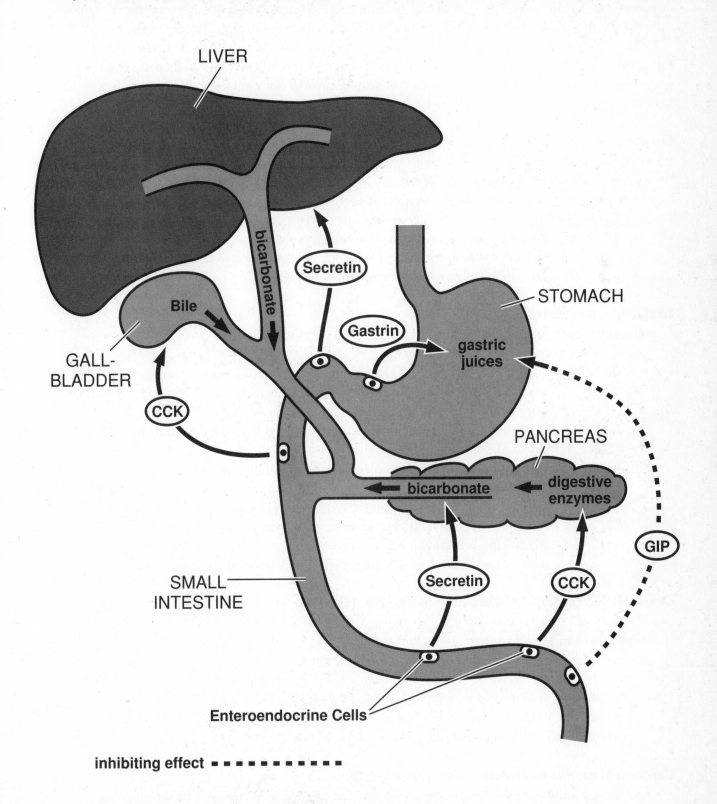

LIVER

bicarbonate

Secretin

Bile

Gastrin

gastric juices

STOMACH

GALL-BLADDER

CCK

PANCREAS

bicarbonate

digestive enzymes

SMALL INTESTINE

Secretin

CCK

GIP

Enteroendocrine Cells

inhibiting effect ▪ ▪ ▪ ▪ ▪ ▪ ▪ ▪

ENDOCRINE TISSUES / Pancreatic Islets

The pancreas is a long, flat, glandular organ that lies behind the stomach. It contains both exocrine and endocrine cells. The exocrine cells (acinar cells) release *digestive enzymes* into the duodenum via the pancreatic duct; the endocrine cells release *hormones* into the bloodstream.

The endocrine portion of the pancreas consists of clusters of cells called pancreatic islets (islets of Langerhans). The pancreatic islets contain 4 distinct types of cells — alpha cells that secrete glucagon, beta cells that secrete insulin, D-cells that secrete growth hormone-inhibiting hormone (somatostatin), and F-cells that secrete pancreatic polypeptide.

Glucagon   secreted by alpha cells
secretion stimulated by : decreased levels of blood glucose.
actions : increases blood glucose levels.
> *body cells :* inhibits the uptake of glucose and amino acids.
> *adipose tissue :* breaks down triglycerides into fatty acids and glycerol (lipolysis).
> *liver :* converts glycogen into glucose (glycogenolysis);
> converts other noncarbohydrates into glucose (gluconeogenesis);
> stimulates the synthesis of ketone bodies (ketones).

Insulin   secreted by beta cells
secretion stimulated by : increased levels of blood glucose.
actions : decreases blood glucose levels.
> *body cells :* stimulates the uptake of glucose and its conversion into glycogen.
> activates enzymes important for glycolysis (glucose used for ATP production);
> stimulates uptake of amino acids and protein synthesis;
> inhibits the enzymes that mediate protein and glycogen catabolism.
> *adipose tissue :* facilitates the uptake of glucose by fat cells;
> stimulates the conversion of glucose into fatty acids (lipogenesis);
> inhibits triglyceride catabolism (inhibits the enzyme lipase);
> promotes fat storage (inhibits utilization of fats for ATP production).
> *liver cells :* stimulates the conversion of glucose into glycogen (glycogenesis);
> inhibits the breakdown of glycogen (glycogenolysis);
> inhibits the conversion of noncarbohydrates into glucose (gluconeogenesis).

Growth Hormone-Inhibiting Hormone (GHIH)   also called *Somatostatin.*
> secreted by delta cells (D-cells)
secretion stimulated by : increased levels of blood glucose, amino acids, and CCK.
actions : inhibits the secretion of insulin and glucagon.
> *pancreas :* inhibits the secretion of insulin, glucagon, and pancreatic digestive enzymes.
> *duodenum :* inhibits the secretion of GIP (gastric inhibitory peptide) and secretin.
> *stomach :* inhibits the secretion of gastrin; inhibits stomach motility and absorption.
> *gallbladder :* inhibits gallbladder contractions.

Pancreatic Polypeptide   secreted by F-cells
secretion stimulated by : meals containing protein; fasting; exercise; low blood glucose.
actions : slows absorption of food; regulates the release of pancreatic digestive enzymes.

PANCREATIC ISLETS
Alpha and Beta Cell secretions (D-cells and F-cells not illustrated)

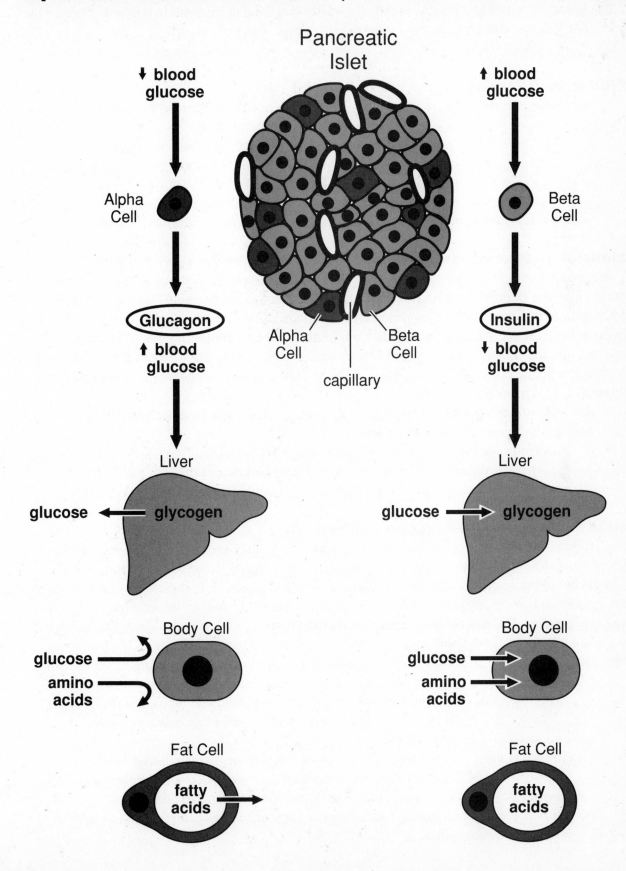

Pancreatic Islet

↓ blood glucose

Alpha Cell

Glucagon

↑ blood glucose

Liver

glucose ← glycogen

Body Cell

glucose

amino acids

Fat Cell

fatty acids

Alpha Cell

Beta Cell

capillary

↑ blood glucose

Beta Cell

Insulin

↓ blood glucose

Liver

glucose → glycogen

Body Cell

glucose

amino acids

Fat Cell

fatty acids

ENDOCRINE TISSUES / Kidneys

The kidneys remove and excrete metabolic wastes and balance electrolyte concentrations in the blood. The kidneys also produce two hormones: erythropoietin and calcitriol.

Erythropoietin   secreted by endocrine cells in the kidneys
  secretion stimulated by : testosterone (basal release of erythropoietin in males);
    decreased oxygen delivery to the kidneys;
    low oxygen due to decreased number of erythrocytes;
    decreased hemoglobin content of erythrocytes;
    decreased blood flow;
    decreased oxygen delivery from lungs to blood.
  action : stimulates increased production of red blood cells in red bone marrow.

Calcitriol (1,25-dihydroxy cholecalciferol or 1,25-dihydroxy vitamin D$_3$)
  The term *vitamin D* refers to a group of closely related chemicals. Ultraviolet light converts a provitamin in the skin into vitamin D$_3$ (also called cholecalciferol); vitamin D$_3$ is carried by the bloodstream to the liver where an enzyme converts it into 25-hydroxycholecalciferol; this chemical formed in the liver is carried by the bloodstream to the proximal tubules of the kidneys where it is converted into the active form of vitamin D (calcitriol). Calcitriol is classified as a hormone because it is produced in the body and is transported in the bloodstream to its target cells. Vitamin D$_3$ (cholecalciferol) is also ingested in the diet.
  activation facilitated by : PTH (low plasma calcium stimulates secretion of PTH).
  action : increases blood calcium levels.
    small intestine : stimulates the active absorption of calcium.
    kidneys : facilitates calcium reabsorption (decreases rate of calcium excretion).
    bone : mobilizes calcium and phosphate out of the bone into the ECF.

Angiotensin II (Renin-Angiotensin Pathway)
  Renin is an enzyme secreted by cells in the kidney in response to low blood pressure in the afferent arterioles, low sodium in the kidney tubules, and sympathetic nerve stimulation.
  In the blood plasma renin activates the plasma protein angiotensin I; angiotensin I is converted into angiotensin II by an enzyme found on the luminal surface of capillary endothelial cells in the lungs. Angiotensin II stimulates the release of aldosterone from the adrenal cortex. So, although renin is not a hormone, it initiates a series of reactions that lead to the secretion of the hormone aldosterone. The overall effect of the renin-angiotensin pathway is to increase the blood pressure.
  secretion stimulated by : low blood pressure in the afferent arterioles of the kidneys;
    low sodium concentrations in the distal tubules of the kidneys;
    sympathetic nerve stimulation of juxtaglomerular cells .
  action : increases blood pressure.
    adrenal glands : stimulates the secretion of aldosterone by the adrenal cortex
        (decreases sodium excretion; increases potassium excretion).
    arterioles : stimulates vasoconstriction (increases resistance to blood flow).
    sympathetic nervous system : stimulates activity of the sympathetic nervous system.
    brain : stimulates thirst.

KIDNEYS

Low blood oxygen stimulates kidney cells to secrete erythropoietin.

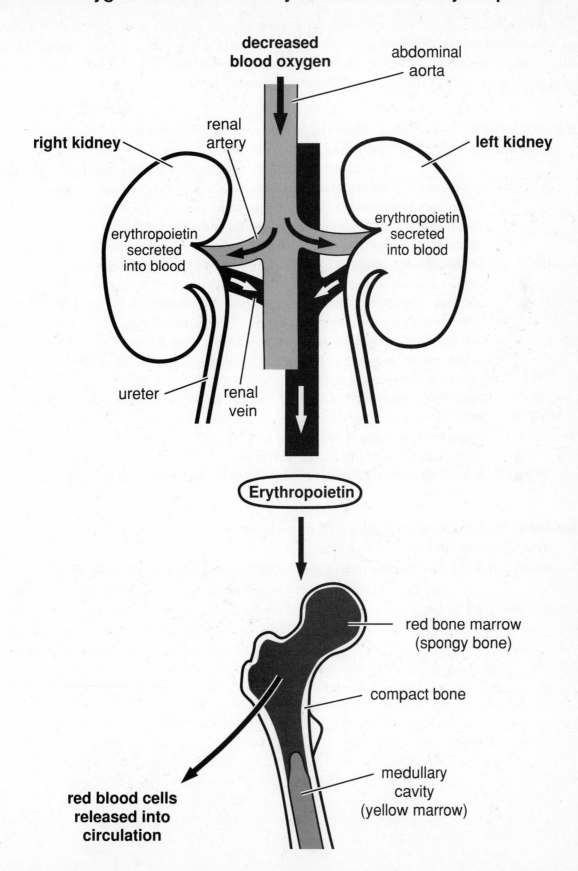

decreased
blood oxygen

abdominal
aorta

right kidney

renal
artery

left kidney

erythropoietin
secreted
into blood

erythropoietin
secreted
into blood

ureter

renal
vein

Erythropoietin

red bone marrow
(spongy bone)

compact bone

**red blood cells
released into
circulation**

medullary
cavity
(yellow marrow)

ENDOCRINE TISSUES / Testes

The principal androgen (male sex hormone) secreted by the testes is testosterone. It is a steroid that is synthesized from cholesterol in the interstitial cells of Leydig; these cells are located between the seminiferous tubules of the testes. In some of its target cells testosterone is not active until it is converted into another androgen called *dihydrotestosterone (DHT)*.

Testosterone   secreted by interstitial endocrinocytes of the testes
   secretion stimulated by : luteinizing hormone (LH);
                                also called interstitial cell-stimulating hormone (ICSH) in males.
   actions :   *stimulates the development of external genitals and accessory organs;*
               stimulates spermatogenesis (sperm production);
               contributes to male sexual behavior and sex drive;
               stimulates protein synthesis (heavier muscle and bone mass);
               stimulates development of secondary sexual characteristics.
               penis : increases in length and width.
               scrotum : becomes pigmented and rugose (wrinkled).
               seminal vesicles : enlarge and secrete fructose-rich fluid.
               prostate and urethral glands : enlarge and secrete fluid.
               vocal cords : increase in length and thickness (lowering of voice).
               larynx (voice box) : enlarges.
               body hair : growth of pubic hair, axillary hair, beard, chest hair, anal hair.
               skeletal muscles : enlarge.
               shoulders : become broader.
               sebaceous glands : increased secretions.
               brain : development of aggressive behavior and interest in the opposite sex.

Inhibin   secreted by sustentacular cells of the testes
   secretion stimulated by : testosterone.
   action : inhibits FSH secretion by gonadotrophs in the anterior pituitary gland.

TESTES

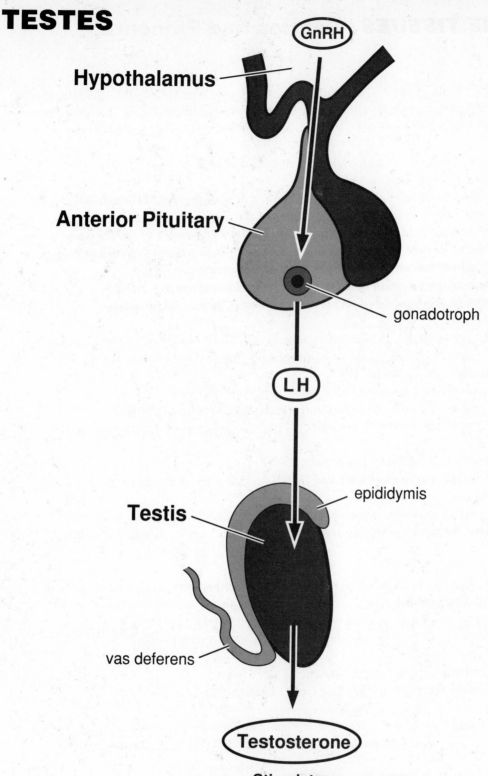

Hypothalamus

Anterior Pituitary

gonadotroph

LH

Testis

epididymis

vas deferens

Testosterone

Stimulates :
development of external genitals
development of accessory reproductive organs
development of secondary sexual characteristics
sperm production (spermatogenesis)
protein synthesis

Contributes to :
male sexual behavior and sex drive

41

ENDOCRINE TISSUES / Ovaries and Placenta

OVARIES

The ovaries are the female gonads. They produce estrogens, progesterone, inhibin, and relaxin. At least six different estrogens have been described; only three are present in significant quantities : beta-estradiol, estrone, and estriol. In nonpregnant women, beta-estradiol is the principal estrogen.

Estrogens   secreted by granulosa / follicle cells of maturing follicles
secretion stimulated by : FSH and LH.
actions : promote the development and maintenance of female reproductive structures;
promote development and maintenance of the secondary sex characteristics;
help control fluid and electrolyte balance; stimulate growth of the breasts;
stimulate protein synthesis; they are synergistic with human growth hormone;
regulate oogenesis (egg development) and the menstrual cycle;
stimulate the secretion of human growth hormone during puberty;
maintain pregnancy and prepare the mammary glands for lactation.

Progesterone   small quantities secreted by follicle cells (follicular phase of menstrual cycle)
large quantities secreted by luteal cells (luteal phase of menstrual cycle)
secretion stimulated by : FSH and LH.
actions : prepares the uterine lining and mammary glands for pregnancy.
uterus : prepares the endometrium (lining of the uterus) for implantation.
breasts : stimulates growth and prepares the mammary glands for milk secretion.

Inhibin   secreted by cells of the corpus luteum
actions : inhibits the secretion of FSH and GnRH (and to a lesser extent LH).

Relaxin   secreted by cells of the corpus luteum during pregnancy
actions : relaxes the pubic symphysis and dilates the uterine cervix, facilitating delivery.

PLACENTA

The placenta is the structure through which materials are exchanged between the fetus and mother.
Estrogens and Progesterone   secreted from the 60th day of pregnancy until birth
actions :   uterus : maintain the lining of the uterus during pregnancy.
mammary glands : prepare the mammary glands to secrete milk.

Inhibin   secreted by cells of the corpus luteum
action : inhibits the secretion of FSH and GnRH (and to a lesser extent LH).

Relaxin   secreted by cells of the chorionic cytotrophoblast and the placental base plate
actions : relaxes the pubic symphysis and dilates the uterine cervix, facilitating delivery.

Human Chorionic Gonadotropin (hCG)   secreted by the chorion of the placenta
action : maintains the activity of the corpus luteum until the 4th month of pregnancy.

Human Chorionic Somatomammotropin (hCS)   secreted by cells of the chorion
actions :   mammary glands : prepares mammary glands for lactation (production of milk);
enhances the growth of the breasts.
body cells : decreases glucose utilization by the mother (makes it available to fetus).
fat cells : promotes release of fatty acids from fat deposits (energy source for mother).

OVARIES

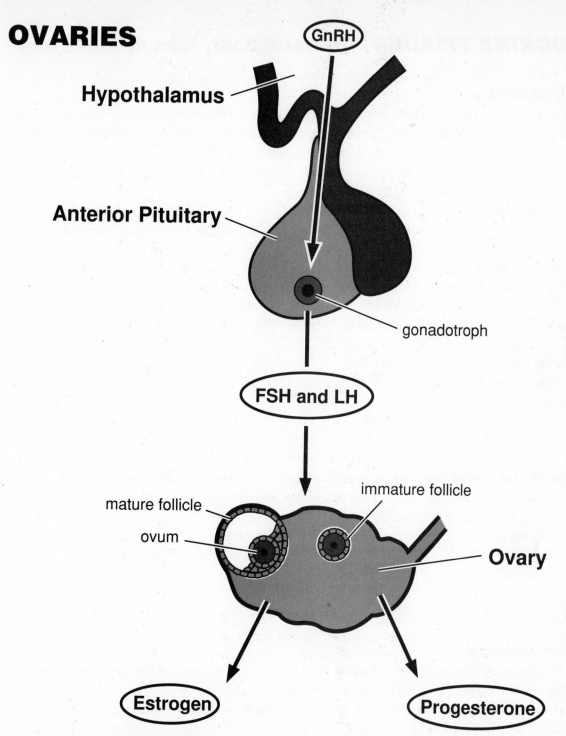

GnRH

Hypothalamus

Anterior Pituitary

gonadotroph

FSH and LH

mature follicle

immature follicle

ovum

Ovary

Estrogen

Progesterone

Stimulates :
protein synthesis
growth of breasts
secretion of hGH during puberty
development of female reproductive structures
development of secondary sexual characteristics

Controls :
the menstrual cycle
fluid and electrolyte balance
egg development (oogenesis)

Prepares
Uterine Lining and Mammary Glands
for Pregnancy

ENDOCRINE TISSUES / Pineal Gland, Heart, and Liver

PINEAL GLAND

The pineal gland (also called the *epiphysis cerebri*) is attached to the roof of the 3rd ventricle in the brain; it is under the posterior end of the corpus callosum and is connected by a stalk to the posterior commissure. It is called pineal because its shape is similar to a pine cone. During the dark period of the day, melatonin synthesis and secretion are increased; during the light period of the day, secretion of melatonin is maintained at a low level.

The secretion of melatonin is regulated by norepinephrine that is released by the postganglionic sympathetic nerves that innervate the pineal gland. The sympathetic nerves that innervate the pineal gland are stimulated by nerve activity that starts in the retina and passes via the hypothalamus (suprachiasmatic nuclei) to the pineal gland. The function of melatonin in humans is unclear.

In other animals the hormone melatonin coordinates internal events with the light-dark cycle in the environment. There is some evidence that melatonin regulates reproductive activities by inhibiting the secretion of gonadotropic hormones. This may affect the sexual behavior of some seasonally breeding animals.

Melatonin   secreted by pinealocytes
secretion stimulated by : darkness (inhibited by light).
actions : unknown

HEART

Atrial Natriuretic Factor   secreted by cardiac muscle fibers of the atria
secretion stimulated by : stretching of cardiac muscle fibers in the atria.
action : lowers blood pressure.
> *kidneys :*   decreases sodium reabsorption by kidneys (increases sodium excretion); inhibits the secretion of renin (decreased levels of angiotensin II);
> *adrenal glands :* inhibits the secretion of aldosterone.

LIVER
Somatomedins

The effects of human growth hormone on the formation of bone, cartilage, and protein metabolism depend on interaction between human growth hormones and somatomedins. Somatomedins are growth factors that are synthesized by liver, cartilage, and many other tissues. Two types of somatomedins are classified as circulating hormones because they travel via the bloodstream to distant target cells; the circulating somatomedins are IGF-I (insulinlike growth factor I) and IGF-II (insulinlike growth factor II).

> *secretion stimulated by :* hGH (Human Growth Hormone).
> *actions :*   *bone :* stimulate bone and body growth.
> *cartilage :* stimulate cartilage growth.

PINEAL GLAND, HEART, and LIVER

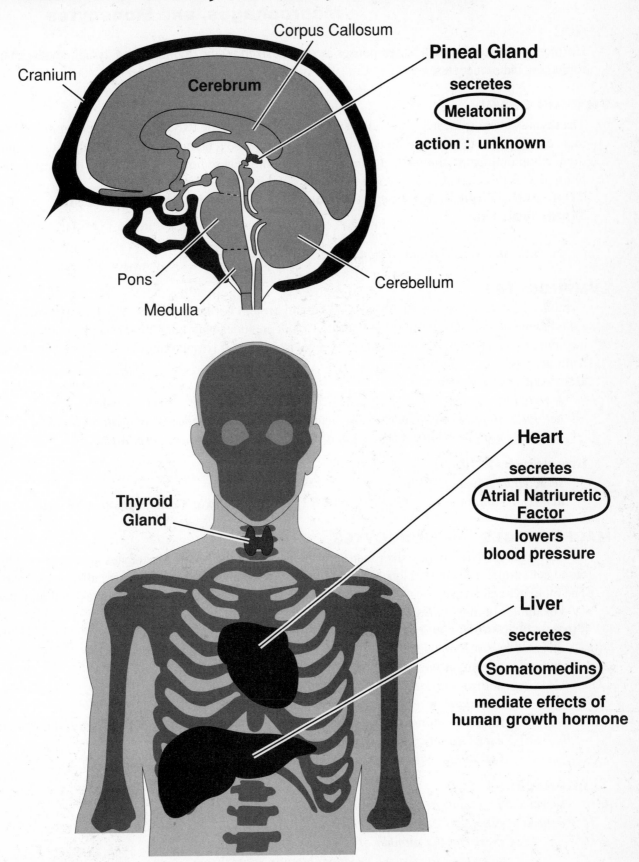

Corpus Callosum

Pineal Gland

secretes

Melatonin

action : unknown

Cranium

Cerebrum

Pons

Medulla

Cerebellum

Heart

secretes

Atrial Natriuretic Factor

lowers blood pressure

Thyroid Gland

Liver

secretes

Somatomedins

mediate effects of human growth hormone

ENDOCRINE TISSUES / Thymus Gland, Lymphocytes, Macrophages, and Monocytes

Hormones that regulate defense responses are synthesized by the thymus gland, lymphocytes, macrophages, and monocytes.

THYMUS GLAND

The thymus gland is located behind the sternum and between the two lungs in the region of the thoracic cavity called the mediastinum. The thymus secretes several hormones, including : thymosin, thymic humoral factor, thymic factor, and thymopoietin. These hormones stimulate the activity of lymphocytes (T cells) after they leave the thymus and migrate to other tissues.

Thymosin, Thymic Humoral Factor (THF), Thymic Factor (TF), and Thymopoietin

secreted by : cells in the thymus gland.

action : stimulate the maturation and activity of T-lymphocytes.

LYMPHOCYTES

Lymphocytes are a type of white blood cell. Small protein hormones secreted by lymphocytes are called *lymphokines*. The more general term *cytokine* includes both lymphokines and monokines (secreted by monocytes and macrophages). Two examples of lymphokines are : gamma interferon and interleukin-2.

Gamma Interferon

secreted by : helper T cells, cytotoxic T cells, and natural killer cells (NK cells).

actions : stimulates phagocytosis by neutrophils and macrophages; activates NK cells; enhances both cellular and antibody-mediated immune responses.

Interleukin-2 (IL-2)

secreted by : helper T cells.

actions : stimulates the proliferation of B cells and cytotoxic T cells; activates NK cells.

MACROPHAGES and MONOCYTES

Macrophages are phagocytic cells found in many tissues of the body. Monocytes are a type of white blood cell. Small protein hormones secreted by macrophages and monocytes are called *monokines*. The more general term *cytokine* includes both lymphokines (secreted by lymphocytes) and monokines. Two examples of monokines are : tumor necrosis factor and interleukin-1.

Tumor Necrosis Factor (TNF)

secreted by : macrophages.

actions : stimulates the accumulation of leukocytes at sites of inflammation; activates inflammatory leukocytes to kill microbes; stimulates macrophages to produce interleukin-1 (IL-1); induces synthesis of colony-stimulating factors by endothelial cells and fibroblasts; exerts an interferonlike protective effect against viruses; acts on the hypothalamus to induce fever.

Interleukin-1 (IL-1)

secreted by : monocytes and macrophages.

actions : stimulates B cell and T cell proliferation; increases the number of circulating neutrophils; stimulates the liver to produce immune substances; acts on the hypothalamus to induce fever.

MACROPHAGES

Microbes ingested by macrophages stimulate the release of Tumor Necrosis Factor (TNF) and Interleukin-1 (IL-1).

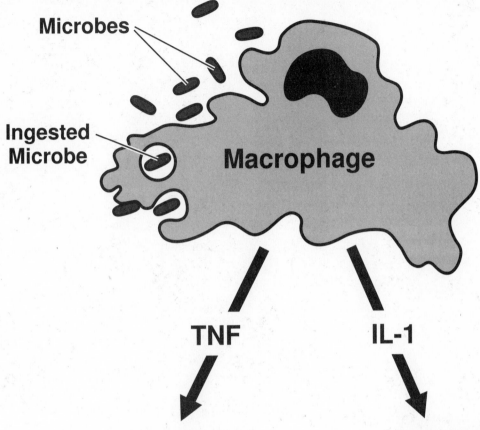

Microbes

Ingested Microbe

Macrophage

TNF

IL-1

Leukocytes

stimulates accumulation at
sites of inflammation

activates leukocytes
to kill microbes

Macrophages

stimulates the synthesis of
IL-1

Endothelial Cells and Fibroblasts

induces the synthesis of
colony-stimulating factors

Body Cells

exerts an antiviral effect

Hypothalamus

induces fever

Lymphocytes

stimulates proliferation
of B cells and T cells

Neutrophils

increases number of
circulating neutrophils

Liver

stimulates production of
immune substances

Hypothalamus

induces fever

3 Endocrine Physiology

ENDOCRINE PHYSIOLOGY / Homeostasis

HOMEOSTASIS and STRESS

Homeostasis   In order to function effectively, the cells in the human body require relatively stable conditions. The relative stability of the internal environment (the extracellular fluid) is called homeostasis (*homeo* = same; *stasis* = standing still). An organism is said to be in homeostasis when its internal environment :
>   (1) contains the optimal concentrations of gases, nutrients, ions, and water;
>   (2) has an optimal temperature; and
>   (3) has an optimal fluid volume.

Stress   Any stimulus that tends to create an imbalance in the internal environment is called a stress. Stresses may originate in the external environment or from within the body. Stresses from the external environment include changes in temperature, loud noises, and insufficient oxygen. Examples of stresses inside the body include changes in blood pressure, in blood calcium level, in blood sugar level, or in blood pH.

Homeostatic Mechanisms   The body has many regulating (homeostatic) mechanisms that oppose the forces of stress and bring the internal environment back into balance. The homeostatic responses of the body are regulated by the nervous and endocrine systems working together or independently. In both the nervous and the endocrine systems, homeostasis is maintained by negative feedback systems.

FEEDBACK SYSTEMS   (Loops)

All important conditions of the internal and external environments are constantly monitored. In a feedback system, information about changes in a particular condition is detected by receptors and fed back (reported) to a control center; the control center determines the appropriate response, which is carried out by effector cells (target cells in the endocrine system).

Negative Feedback (maintains homeostasis)
In a negative feedback system the response reverses (has a negative effect on) the original stimulus; thus, a negative feedback system tends to maintain homeostasis.

Positive Feedback
In a positive feedback system the response enhances the original stimulus. Labor contractions are an example of positive feedback. Contractions stimulate more contractions.

CONTROL OF HORMONAL SECRETIONS

Types of Input
The secretion of hormones by endocrine cells is controlled by 3 basic types of input :
>   (1) Other Hormones (Tropic Hormones)
>   (2) Chemical Changes in the Blood
>   (3) Signals from the Nervous System

Regulation of Secretion
Negative feedback systems prevent overproduction or underproduction of hormones. For example, low blood calcium levels stimulate the release of PTH from parathyroid glands, and the PTH stimulates the release of calcium from bone tissue, returning blood calcium levels to normal. Normal blood calcium levels inhibit the secretion of PTH, stopping the response.

CONTROL OF HORMONE SECRETION
Negative Feedback

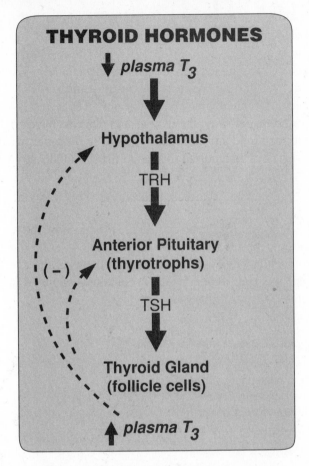

THYROID HORMONES

↓ *plasma T$_3$*

↓

Hypothalamus

TRH

↓

Anterior Pituitary
(thyrotrophs)

TSH

↓

Thyroid Gland
(follicle cells)

↑ *plasma T$_3$*

(–)

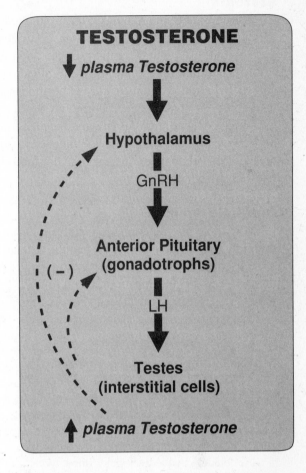

TESTOSTERONE

↓ *plasma Testosterone*

↓

Hypothalamus

GnRH

↓

Anterior Pituitary
(gonadotrophs)

LH

↓

Testes
(interstitial cells)

↑ *plasma Testosterone*

(–)

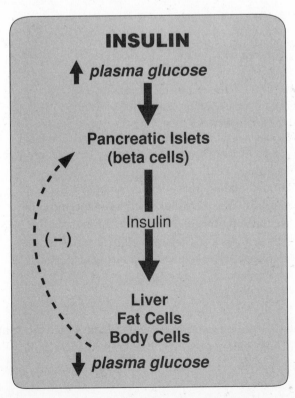

INSULIN

↑ *plasma glucose*

↓

Pancreatic Islets
(beta cells)

Insulin

↓

Liver
Fat Cells
Body Cells

↓ *plasma glucose*

(–)

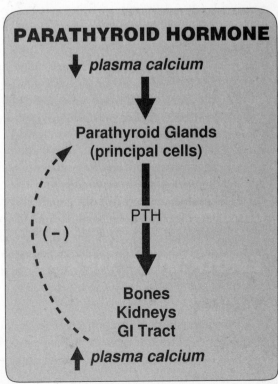

PARATHYROID HORMONE

↓ *plasma calcium*

↓

Parathyroid Glands
(principal cells)

PTH

↓

Bones
Kidneys
GI Tract

↑ *plasma calcium*

(–)

51

ENDOCRINE PHYSIOLOGY / Hormone Synthesis

Steroids

All steroid hormones are derived from *cholesterol*. Steroid hormones are produced by the adrenal cortex (aldosterone, cortisol, androgens, estrogen), the testes (testosterone), the ovaries (estrogen and progesterone), and the placenta (estrogen and progesterone).

All steroid hormones are slight modifications of the cholesterol molecule. The same biochemical pathways for the synthesis of steroid hormones are present in each of the endocrine glands mentioned above; they produce different hormones because they have different enzyme concentrations. The testes have high concentrations of enzymes needed for the testosterone pathway; the ovaries and placenta have high concentrations of the enzymes needed to transform testosterone into estrogen; the cells in the outer two layers of the adrenal cortex have high concentrations of the enzymes required for the cortisol and aldosterone pathways.

Biogenic Amines

All amine hormones are derived from the amino acid *tyrosine*. Amine hormones are produced by the thyroid gland (thyroid hormone) and the adrenal medulla (epinephrine and norepinephrine).

Thyroid Hormones Triiodothyronine (T_3) and thyroxine (T_4) are synthesized in the follicles of the thyroid gland by attaching iodine to tyrosine. T_3 contains 3 atoms of iodine, while T_4 contains 4 atoms of iodine; this is the only difference between the two molecules.

The synthesis of thyroid hormones includes the following steps:

(1) Iodide Trapping Iodide (I^-) is actively transported from the blood into follicular cells.

(2) Thyroglobulin (TGB) Synthesis A large glycoprotein is synthesized by follicular cells.
It contains more than 100 tyrosine residues, a few of which become iodinated.
TGBs are packaged in secretory vesicles and released into the lumen of the follicle.

(3) Iodide Oxidation Peroxidase catalyzes the conversion of iodide to iodine (I_2).
As iodide ions are being oxidized they pass into the lumen of the follicle.

(4) Tyrosine Iodination Iodine attaches to some tyrosines that are part of the TGB molecules.
Binding one iodine yields monoiodotyrosine (T_1);
binding two iodines yields diiodotyrosine (T_2).

(5) T_1 and T_2 Coupling
Joining two molecules of T_2 forms T_4 (thyroxine).
joining one molecule of T_2 with one of T_1 forms T_3 (triiodothyronine).

(6) Colloid Pinocytosis Colloid droplets re-enter follicular cells and merge with lysosomes.
Enzymes cleave off molecules of T_3 and T_4.

(7) Thyroid Hormone Secretion In response to TSH, T_3 and T_4 are released into the blood.

(8) Thyroid Hormone Blood Transport T_3 and T_4 combine with a transport protein called thyroxine-binding globulin (TBG), making them soluble in the watery blood plasma.

(9) Thyroid Hormone Action Both T_3 and T_4 are secreted by the thyroid gland, but most of the T_4 is converted into T_3 when it reaches the target cells. T_3 binds with receptors in the nuclei of target cells. Specific genes are activated, resulting in the synthesis of a number of different enzymes.

Epinephrine and Norepinephrine The cells of the adrenal medulla that secrete epinephrine and norepinephrine are modified postganglionic sympathetic neurons. They are classified as endocrine cells because they secrete their chemicals into the blood and alter the activities of target cells throughout the body. The amino acid tyrosine is actively transported into these cells and transformed by a series of enzymatically controlled reactions into norepinephrine and epinephrine. The sequence is: tyrosine, dopa, dopamine, norepinephrine, and finally epinephrine.

Peptides

Most peptides are synthesized as parts of prohormones. *Prohormones* are large peptides, which are split by enzymes to form fragments that are active hormones. The hormones that result from the cleavage of prohormones are stored in secretory vesicles.

THYROID HORMONES
Synthesis and Action

key :

TGB = Thyroglobulin
TSH = Thyroid-Stimulating Hormone
TBG = Thyroxine-Binding Globulin

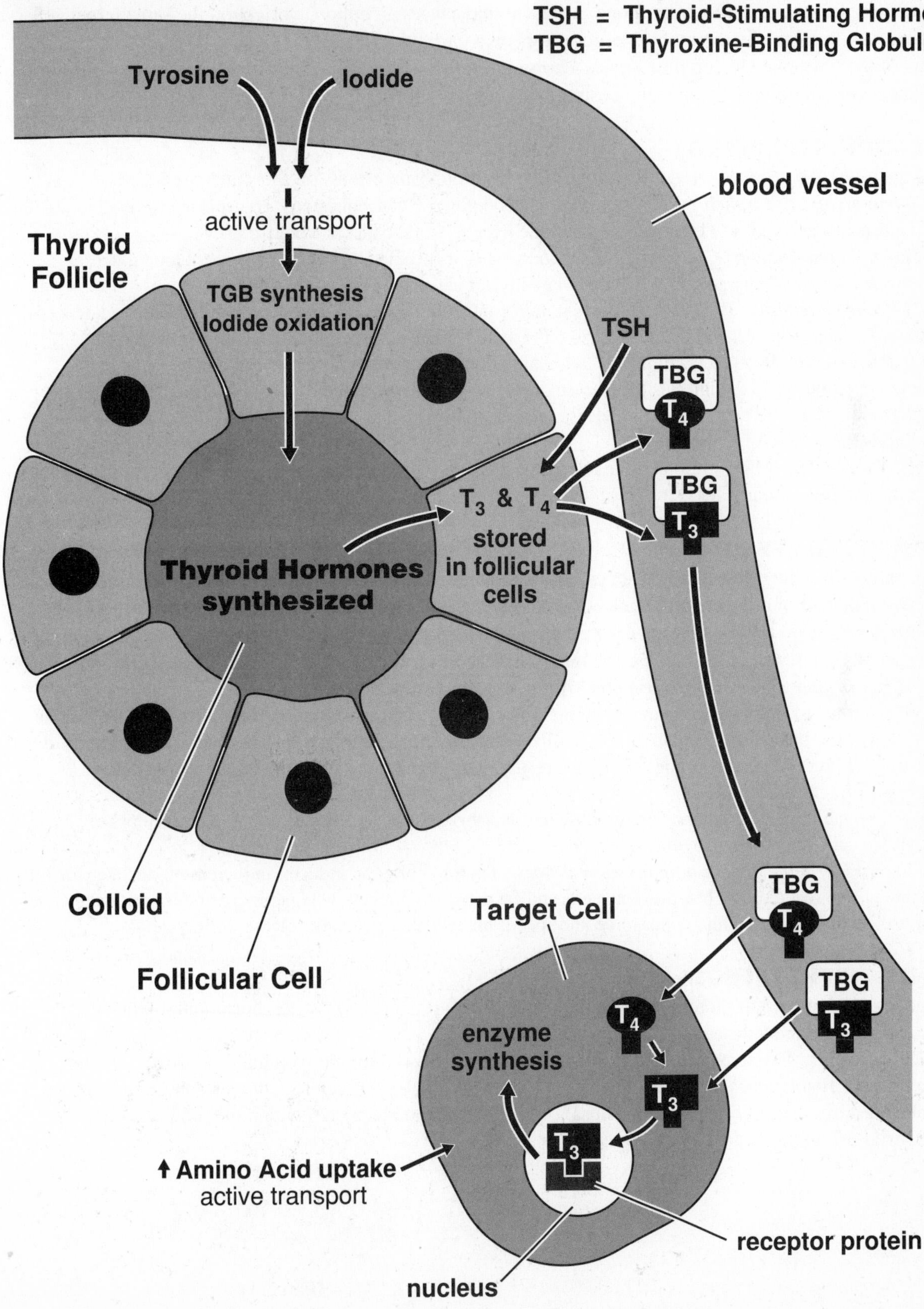

Tyrosine   Iodide

blood vessel

active transport

Thyroid Follicle

TGB synthesis
Iodide oxidation

TSH

TBG
T_4

TBG
T_3

T_3 & T_4
stored
in follicular
cells

Thyroid Hormones synthesized

TBG
T_4

Colloid

Target Cell

TBG
T_3

Follicular Cell

T_4

enzyme
synthesis

T_3

T_3

↑ **Amino Acid uptake**
active transport

receptor protein

nucleus

ENDOCRINE PHYSIOLOGY / Hormone Interactions

The effects of hormones on their target cells may be altered by a variety of factors. The effects of a hormone are lessened if another hormone is present that causes an opposite effect on the same target cells. If there is some change in the number of receptors on a particular type of target cell, it will alter the effects of the hormone. In certain cases two hormones must act on the same target organ in sequence or simultaneously in order to achieve the desired response.

ANTAGONISTIC EFFECT

Antagonistic hormones are two hormones that have opposite effects on the same target cells.

Glucagon and Epinephrine   Glucagon raises blood glucose concentrations; epinephrine lowers blood glucose concentrations. The target cells include liver cells, fat cells, and body cells.

Glucagon and Insulin   Glucagon raises blood glucose concentrations; insulin lowers blood glucose concentrations. The target cells include liver cells, fat cells, and body cells.

PTH and Calcitonin   PTH raises blood calcium concentrations; calcitonin lowers blood calcium concentrations. The target cells of calcitonin and PTH include bone cells and kidney cells.

GHRH and GHIH   GHRH stimulates the release of human growth hormone by somatotrophs in the anterior pituitary; GHIH inhibits the release of human growth hormone.

PRH and PIH   PRH stimulates the release of prolactin by lactotrophs in the anterior pituitary; PIH inhibits the release of prolactin.

MRH and MIH   MRH stimulates the release of melanocyte-stimulating hormone (MSH) by corticotrophs in the anterior pituitary; MIH inhibits the release of MSH.

PERMISSIVE EFFECT

In this interaction the effect of a hormone on its target cell is enhanced by another hormone. When previous exposure of a target cell to one hormone enhances its responsiveness to a second hormone, the first hormone is said to have a permissive effect on the target cell. The increased sensitivity of the target cell is usually the result of an increased number of receptors for the second hormone (up-regulation).

Estrogens alter Progesterone receptors   An increase in estrogens induces an increase in the number of progesterone receptors on cells in the uterine lining. Both estrogens and progesterone prepare the uterine lining for the possible implantation of a fertilized egg. In the female reproductive cycle, the secretion of estrogens precedes that of progesterone; the resulting up-regulation causes the progesterone to have a greater effect.

Estrogens alter LH receptors   An increase in estrogens induces an increase in the LH receptors on ovarian cells; this triggers ovulation.

Thyroid Hormone alters Epinephrine receptors   Thyroid hormone induces an increase in the number of epinephrine receptors on heart muscle cells and fat cells. As a result, when epinephrine is secreted, heart muscle cells contract with greater force and speed; fat cells increase their release of fatty acids.

SYNERGISTIC EFFECT

In this interaction, two or more hormones are needed for full expression of the hormonal effects; each hormone complements the action of the other hormone.

LH and FSH   The combined effects of LH and FSH are needed for the secretion of estrogens by the ovaries. LH stimulates theca cells (which surround the follicles) to secrete androgens; the androgens are absorbed by adjacent follicular (granulosa) cells. FSH activates enzymes within the follicular cells that convert the androgens into estrogen.

ANTAGONISTIC HORMONES

Insulin : stimulates the conversion of glucose to glycogen (uptake of glucose).

Glucagon : stimulates the conversion of glycogen to glucose (release of glucose).

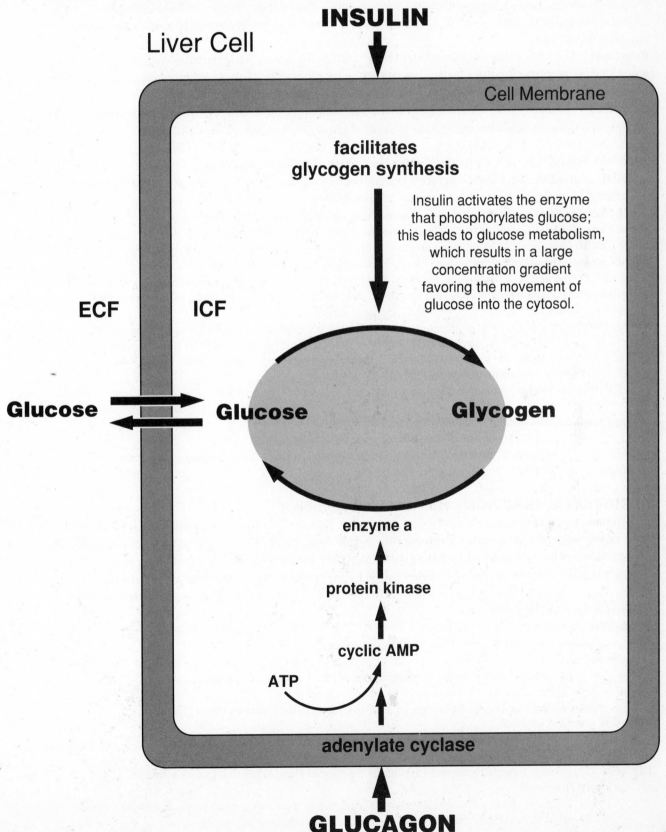

INSULIN

Liver Cell

Cell Membrane

**facilitates
glycogen synthesis**

Insulin activates the enzyme that phosphorylates glucose; this leads to glucose metabolism, which results in a large concentration gradient favoring the movement of glucose into the cytosol.

ECF   ICF

Glucose   **Glucose**   **Glycogen**

enzyme a

protein kinase

cyclic AMP

ATP

adenylate cyclase

GLUCAGON

ENDOCRINE PHYSIOLOGY / Stress Response

General Adaptation Syndrome (GAS)   The response to stress is called the general adaptation syndrome.
Stressors   The many types of stimuli that trigger the stress response are called stressors. Physical stimuli include prolonged heavy exercise, physical trauma, shock (blood loss), decreased blood oxygen, poisons, bacterial toxins, prolonged exposure to cold, and pain. Emotional or psychological stimuli include fear, anxiety, and anger.
Responses   The body responds immediately by activating the sympathetic nervous system; a slower but longer lasting response involves the actions of certain hormones : cortisol, aldosterone, epinephrine, human growth hormone, and thyroid hormone.
Exhaustion   Exhaustion is caused mainly by loss of potassium (cells dehydrate), depletion of cortisol (blood sugar levels drop), and weakened organs. If stress is too great, it may lead to death.

ALARM REACTION   Sympathetic Nervous System Response

Activation of the sympathetic nervous system is often referred to as the fight-or-flight response. Major effects of <u>increased</u> general sympathetic activity include:

Heart   An increased rate and strength of contraction increase cardiac output and blood pressure.
Blood Vessels   Blood is shunted from skin and internal organs to the skeletal muscles.
Blood Clot Mechanism   The blood clots faster.
Blood Volume   The spleen releases stored blood, increasing blood volume and blood pressure.
Blood Cell Production   The red bone marrow is stimulated to increase blood cell production.
Lung Ventilation   Respiratory muscles are stimulated and bronchioles (air passageways) dilate, increasing lung ventilation.
Energy Production   In the liver, glycogen is converted into glucose, which is released into the blood; glucose is synthesized from noncarbohydrates and released into the blood. In adipose tissue triglycerides are broken down into glycerol and fatty acids (energy sources), which are released into the blood. Glucose, fatty acids, and glycerol are used for ATP production.
Skin   The arrector pili muscles contract (goose pimples); sweat glands secrete sweat.
Eyes   The pupils dilate.
Adrenal Medulla   The adrenal medulla is stimulated to release epinephrine and norepinephrine, which prepare many organs for fight-or-flight.
Inhibition of "Nonessential" Systems :   Activities of the digestive, urinary, reproductive, and immune systems are inhibited.

RESISTANCE REACTION   Hormonal Response

The resistance reaction is slower to start, but longer lasting. The hypothalamus receives input from all areas of the brain and all sensory receptors of the body. Regardless of the origin of the stress stimulus, the hypothalamic neurons that secrete CRH, GHRH, and TRH are stimulated. These releasing hormones are secreted into the primary plexus and carried by the hypophyseal portal veins to the secondary plexus in the anterior pituitary where they trigger the release of ACTH, hGH, and TSH. The effects of these anterior pituitary hormones are as follows :

(1) ACTH (Adrenocorticotropic Hormone)
Stimulates the adrenal cortex to secrete aldosterone and cortisol.
Aldosterone
Decreases water excretion by the kidneys; increases blood volume and blood pressure.
Cortisol
Stimulates the conversion of glycogen to glucose by liver cells; increases blood glucose levels.
(2) hGH (Human Growth Hormone)
fat cells : stimulates catabolism of triglycerides; stimulates release of fatty acids and glycerol into the blood.
liver : stimulates the conversion of glycogen to glucose; increases blood glucose levels.
(3) TSH (Thyroid-Stimulating Hormone)   Stimulates the thyroid gland to secrete thyroid hormones.
Thyroid Hormones
heart : increase the rate and strength of contraction, which increases cardiac output and blood pressure.
body cells : increase the metabolic rate (the rate of ATP production increased).

STRESS RESPONSE (General Adaptation Syndrome)

Stress

Hypothalamus

Alarm Reaction
Sympathetic Nervous System

Resistance Reaction
Hypothalamic Hormones

CRH
GHRH
TRH

Visceral Effectors

fight-or-flight response

Spleen
stored blood released

Bone
increased blood cell production

Liver
glycogenolysis

Skin
sweating
arrector pili muscles contract

Heart
increased cardiac output

Blood vessels
blood shunted to skeletal muscles

Blood
clots faster

Lungs
increased ventilation

Nonessential Systems
inhibited

Adrenal Medulla

effects of epinephrine supplement and prolong fight-or-flight response

Anterior Pituitary

hGH ACTH TSH

Liver
↑ glycogenolysis

Adipose Tissue
↑ lipolysis

Adrenal Cortex

Cortisol   Aldosterone

Thyroid Gland

TH

Liver
↑ amino acid uptake
↑ gluconeogenesis

Muscle
↑ protein catabolism

Adipose Tissue
↑ lipolysis

Blood Vessels
↑ vasoconstriction

Immune System
↓ inflammation

Heart
↑ cardiac output
↑ blood pressure

Body Cells
↑ metabolic rate
↑ ATP production

Kidneys
↑ sodium retention
↑ blood pressure

ENDOCRINE PHYSIOLOGY / Nutrient and Ion Balance

The plasma concentrations of nutrients and major ions are maintained at relatively constant levels by the homeostatic actions of hormones.

Glucose   (Insulin, Cortisol, Epinephrine, Glucagon, Human Growth Hormone, and Thyroid Hormones)

The normal plasma glucose concentration is about 70 mg / dL. The blood glucose level at any given time depends upon the balance between the amount of glucose entering the bloodstream and the amount leaving it. Glucose enters the bloodstream primarily from the intestine (dietary intake) and from the liver (conversion of glycogen into glucose); glucose leaves the bloodstream as it enters body cells to be used for energy production and as it enters the liver to be stored as glycogen.   At least 6 hormones are involved in the regulation of blood glucose concentration: insulin, cortisol, epinephrine, glucagon, human growth hormone, and thyroid hormones.

Calcium   (Parathyroid Hormone, Calcitriol, and Calcitonin)

The normal plasma calcium concentration is about 10 mg / dL. Nearly all of the body calcium is in the bones (99%). Calcium ions act as second messengers, and are necessary for blood coagulation, muscle contraction, and nerve function.   There are 3 principal hormones that regulate the plasma concentration of calcium ions : parathyroid hormone (PTH), calcitriol, and calcitonin.

PTH increases plasma calcium by stimulating bone *resorption* (release of calcium from the bones), by increasing the *reabsorption* (return of calcium from kidney tubules to the blood) of calcium in the kidneys, and by stimulating *absorption* of dietary calcium in the intestine.

Calcitriol increases plasma calcium by increasing the *reabsorption* of calcium by the kidneys and by stimulating *absorption* of dietary calcium in the intestine.

Calcitonin decreases plasma calcium by inhibiting bone *resorption* and by increasing the excretion of calcium by the kidneys.

Phosphorus   (PTH and Calcitriol)

Nearly all of the phosphorus in the body is located in the bones (85 to 90%). The normal plasma phosphorus concentration is about 12 mg / dL. Two hormones are responsible for keeping the plasma phosphorus levels constant: PTH and calcitriol.

PTH decreases the plasma phosphorus by inhibiting the *reabsorption* of phosphorus in the kidneys.

Calcitriol increases the plasma phosphorus by stimulating the *absorption* of dietary phosphorus in the intestine.

Sodium   (Aldosterone)

Most of the sodium in the body is located in bones and cartilage. Only 11.2% of the total body sodium is present in the plasma. When the plasma sodium concentration decreases, aldosterone is released, enhancing the reabsorption of sodium by the kidneys.

Potassium   (Aldosterone)

Most of the potassium in the body is inside the cells (89.6 % is intracellular). Only about 0.4% of the total potassium in the body is in the plasma. When plasma potassium levels rise, aldosterone increases the tubular secretion of potassium into the lumens of the kidney tubules; excess potassium is excreted in urine.

Hydrogen Ions (pH)   (Aldosterone)

The normal pH of the blood is 7.4. When the pH falls below 7.4 the condition is called *acidosis*; when it rises above 7.4, the condition is called *alkalosis*. The pH of urine varies from 4.5 to 8.0. As blood plasma becomes more acidic, aldosterone increases the tubular secretion of hydrogen ions into the lumens of the kidney tubules; excess hydrogen ions are excreted in urine.

CALCIUM BALANCE
Calcium homeostasis is regulated by
Parathyroid Hormone (PTH), Calcitriol, and Calcitonin

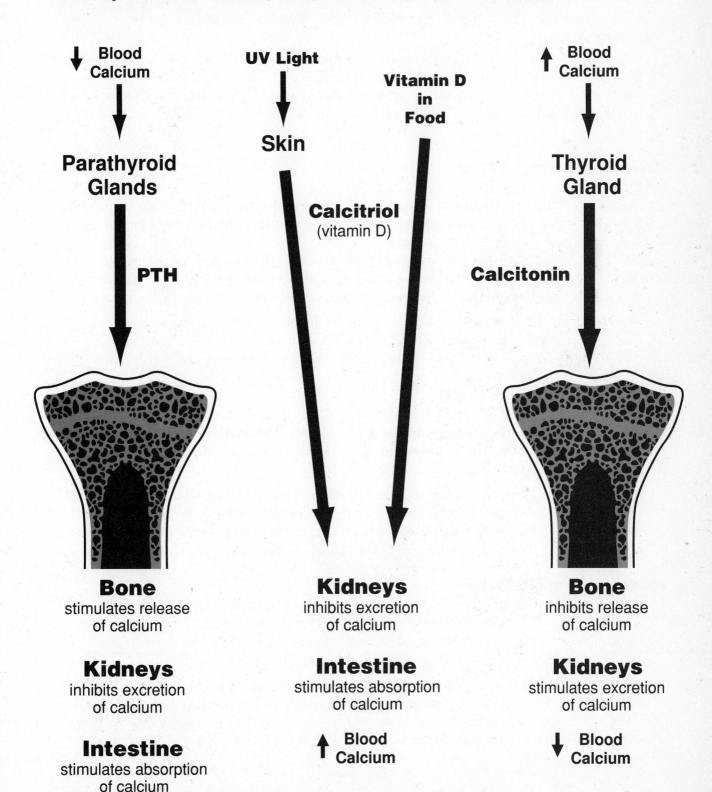

↓ **Blood Calcium**

UV Light

Vitamin D in Food

↑ **Blood Calcium**

Skin

Parathyroid Glands

Thyroid Gland

Calcitriol
(vitamin D)

PTH

Calcitonin

Bone
stimulates release
of calcium

Kidneys
inhibits excretion
of calcium

Bone
inhibits release
of calcium

Kidneys
inhibits excretion
of calcium

Intestine
stimulates absorption
of calcium

Kidneys
stimulates excretion
of calcium

Intestine
stimulates absorption
of calcium

↑ **Blood Calcium**

↓ **Blood Calcium**

↑ **Blood Calcium**

ENDOCRINE PHYSIOLOGY / Hormone Disorders

Human Growth Hormone (hGH)

hyposecretion *(dwarfism)* Insufficient secretion of growth hormone during childhood leads to a type of dwarfism. Body proportions and mental development are normal.

hypersecretion
childhood (giantism) Oversecretion of growth hormone during childhood leads to giantism. Body proportions and mental development are normal.
adulthood (acromegaly) If oversecretion occurs after long bone growth has ended, the result is a condition called acromegaly. The lower jaw, supraorbital ridges, hands, and feet are noticeably enlarged.

Thyroid Hormones (T₃ and T₄)

hyposecretion
childhood (cretinism) Undersecretion of thyroid hormones during childhood results in a condition called cretinism. Symptoms include stunted growth, mental retardation, sluggishness, dry skin, scanty hair, and low body temperature.
adulthood (myxedema) Undersecretion of thyroid hormones during adulthood results in a condition called myxedema. Symptoms include physical and mental sluggishness, puffiness of the face, obesity, dry skin, fatigue, low body temperature. Mental retardation does <u>not</u> occur.

hypersecretion *(Grave's Disease)* Oversecretion of thyroid hormones results in Grave's disease. Symptoms include an elevated basal metabolic rate, rapid heart rate, increased pulse pressure, restlessness, enlarged thyroid gland, overeating, heat intolerance, and weight loss.

Parathyroid Hormone (PTH)

hyposecretion *(muscle spasms)* Undersecretion of PTH causes reduced activity of osteoclasts in the bones, which leads to decreased blood calcium levels. Symptoms include an abnormally excitable nervous system that fires spontaneously, causing muscle spasms (tetany). Spasms in respiratory muscles can lead to respiratory failure.

hypersecretion *(kidney stones, fragile bones)* Oversecretion of PTH stimulates excessive activity of osteoclasts in the bones; excessive amounts of calcium and phosphate are released into the ECF, causing the bones to become soft, fragile, and subject to spontaneous fracture. Excess calcium and phosphate may form crystals of salts called kidney stones in the urinary tract.

Aldosterone and Cortisol

hyposecretion *(Addison's Disease)* Undersecretion of aldosterone and cortisol results in Addison's disease. Symptoms include decreased blood sodium, increased blood potassium, low blood glucose (hypoglycemia), low blood pressure, increased skin pigmentation, weakened muscles, lessened ability to cope with stress, increased susceptibility to infection.

hypersecretion *(Cushing's Syndrome)* Oversecretion of cortisol and aldosterone results in Cushing's syndrome. Symptoms include high blood glucose (hyperglycemia); decreased blood potassium levels, which interferes with heart and nervous system activities; abnormal retention of water and sodium, which causes edema and high blood pressure; and changes in carbohydrate and protein metabolism.

HORMONE DISORDERS

Disorders	Hormones and Symptoms
Dwarfism	**Human Growth Hormone** (undersecretion during childhood) small body size; normal proportions
Giantism	**Human Growth Hormone** (oversecretion during childhood) large body size; normal proportions
Acromegaly	**Human Growth Hormone** (oversecretion in adulthood) enlarged feet, hands, and jaw
Cretinism	**Thyroid Hormones** (undersecretion during childhood) stunted growth; mental retardation
Myxedema	**Thyroid Hormones** (undersecretion during adulthood) mental sluggishness; dry skin; fatigue
Grave's Disease	**Thyroid Hormones** (oversecretion) increased metabolic rate and heart rate
Muscle Spasms	**Parathyroid Hormone** (undersecretion) abnormally excitable nervous system
Kidney Stones	**Parathyroid Hormone** (oversecretion) calcium phosphate crystals in urinary tract
Addison's Disease	**Aldosterone and Cortisol** (undersecretion) low blood glucose and blood pressure; increased susceptibility to infection
Cushing's Syndrome	**Aldosterone and Cortisol** (oversecretion) high blood glucose and blood pressure; altered protein and carbohydrate metabolism

Diabetes Insipidus   (undersecretion of ADH)

Undersecretion of antidiuretic hormone (ADH) causes a condition known as diabetes insipidus. In the absence of ADH, the walls of the renal tubules in the kidneys remain relatively impermeable to water. As a result very little water is reabsorbed from the urine as it passes through the distal tubules and collecting ducts; the blood volume decreases, and the volume of urine increases. Excessive urine production of up to 25 to 30 liters per day decreases plasma volume, lowering the blood pressure. The dilute urine is tasteless (*insipidus* = tasteless).

Diabetes Mellitus   (undersecretion of insulin)

Undersecretion of insulin causes a condition known as diabetes mellitus. Insulin is required for the uptake of glucose by body cells, especially muscle cells and fat cells. In the absence of insulin the uptake of glucose by these cells is impaired.

Hyperglycemia   The glucose that would normally enter muscle cells and fat cells remains in the blood plasma, causing an increase in blood glucose levels, a condition called hyperglycemia. The liver responds to this condition by converting stored glycogen to glucose, which increases the blood glucose levels even more.

Glycosuria   When the concentrations of glucose become too high, the renal processes that normally return glucose to the blood cannot handle the load, and glucose appears in the urine, a condition called glycosuria.

Osmotic Diuresis   The high concentrations of glucose in the urine raise the osmotic pressure of the urine, creating a hypertonic urine; this diminishes the osmotic pressure gradient between the urine in the collecting duct and the interstitial fluid in the interstitium of the kidney. As a result, less water and electrolytes are reabsorbed and there is an increased excretion of water and electrolytes; this is called osmotic diuresis or polyuria. Because of the presence of glucose, the urine has a sweet taste (*mellitus* = honey). In diabetes mellitus the elevated blood glucose levels are of no use to cells, since glucose cannot enter in the absence of insulin; for this reason diabetes mellitus is often referred to as "starvation in the midst of plenty." The glucose that enters cells under normal conditions is used in the Krebs cycle to produce energy (ATP). In the absence of available glucose the body calls on the fuel reserves present in protein and fat.

Protein Catabolism   Muscle protein is broken down to form amino acids, which are carried to the liver by the bloodstream and converted into glucose; a by-product of deamination is urea. As a result, both glucose and urea are released by the liver into the blood. The ultimate excretion of this urea leads to a loss of nitrogen from the body (negative nitrogen balance); the added glucose increases the blood glucose levels and makes the condition worse. Another negative aspect of the process is the breakdown of muscle tissue (muscle wasting).

Fat Catabolism   Stored fats (triglycerides) are converted into fatty acids, which are released into the circulation and taken up by body cells for the production of ATP (this is referred to as fat mobilization).

Acidosis   The production of ATP from fatty acids produces as a by-product large quantities of acetyl coenzyme A (acetyl CoA); this substance is taken up by the liver and converted into ketones, which are acidic. So the use of fats in large quantities as a substitute fuel results in the release of ketones (ketone bodies) into the blood (this is called ketosis). Since ketones are acidic, the pH of the blood drops, creating a condition called acidosis. In extreme acidosis, sodium and potassium are lost in the urine.

Extreme thirst, hunger, and weight loss are also characteristic of diabetes mellitus.

DIABETES MELLITUS

Insulin Deficiency (glucagon excess)

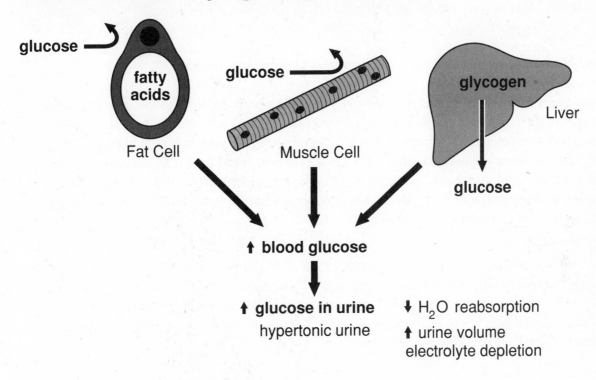

glucose

fatty acids

Fat Cell

glucose

Muscle Cell

glycogen

Liver

glucose

↑ blood glucose

↑ glucose in urine
hypertonic urine

↓ H₂O reabsorption
↑ urine volume
electrolyte depletion

Metabolism of Noncarbohydrates

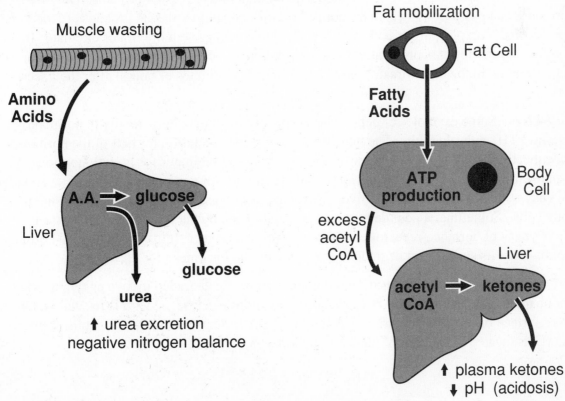

Muscle wasting

Amino Acids

Liver

A.A. → glucose

glucose

urea

↑ urea excretion
negative nitrogen balance

Fat mobilization

Fat Cell

Fatty Acids

ATP production

Body Cell

excess acetyl CoA

Liver

acetyl CoA → ketones

↑ plasma ketones
↓ pH (acidosis)

ENDOCRINE PHYSIOLOGY / Hormone Elimination

A hormone continues to act on its target cells until it is chemically altered by enzymes (mostly in the liver) or excreted by the kidneys.

Bound Hormones : Steroid Hormones and Thyroid Hormones

Steroid Hormones

Steroids are lipids, and are therefore poorly soluble in water. In order to dissolve an effective amount of a steroid hormone in the water-based plasma, it must be bound to protein, which makes it water soluble. It is more difficult to metabolize and excrete bound hormones, so they remain active in the circulation for longer periods of time. The steroid hormones include estrogen, progesterone, testosterone, aldosterone, and cortisol. All of these steroids are degraded by enzymes in the liver. The products of hormone degradation are released into the circulation and excreted by the kidneys.

Thyroid Hormones

Thyroid hormone is classified as a biogenic amine, but it is also bound to plasma protein during transport in the bloodstream. Less than 1% of plasma thyroid hormone is free. The thyroid hormones, triiodothyronine (T_3) and thyroxine (T_4), are deactivated by removal of iodine (deiodination). The enzymes responsible for deactivation of thyroid hormones are located in the liver, the kidneys, and many other tissues.

"Free" Hormones : Peptides, Proteins, and Catecholamines

Free hormones are transported in the bloodstream unbound to plasma proteins. Only free hormones can pass through capillary pores; hormones bound to plasma proteins are too large. Epinephrine, norepinephrine, and most of the peptide and protein hormones circulate "free." For this reason they are comparatively easy to excrete or degrade by enzymes. These hormones remain in the bloodstream for only brief periods (minutes or hours) after their secretion.

Half-Lives
Some examples of peptide hormones are glucagon, human growth hormone, insulin, PTH, and calcitonin. The half-life (the time after secretion for half of the hormones to be inactivated) is about 5-10 minutes for glucagon, 6-20 minutes for growth hormone, 5 minutes for insulin, 20 minutes for PTH, and 10 minutes for calcitonin. All of these peptides are enzymatically degraded in the liver. Some are also degraded in the kidneys and in other body cells. Sometimes a peptide hormone is metabolized by the cells upon which it acts. Endocytosis of hormone-receptor complexes enables a target cell to clear a peptide hormone rapidly from its surface and degrade it with intracellular enzymes.

Degrading Enzymes
Epinephrine and norepinephrine are degraded by two enzymes: MAO (monoamine oxidase) and COMT (catechol-O-methyltransferase). MAO is located on the outer surface of the mitochondria, especially in nerve endings that secrete norepinephrine; COMT is located in the cells of the liver and kidneys.

HORMONE ELIMINATION

Bound Hormones

circulate in the blood
bound to plasma proteins

difficult to metabolize
remain active for hours

Steroids

Thyroid Hormones

"Free" Hormones

circulate "free" in the plasma
(unbound to plasma proteins)

easy to metabolize
inactivated in minutes

Epinephrine

Norepinephrine

Peptide Hormones

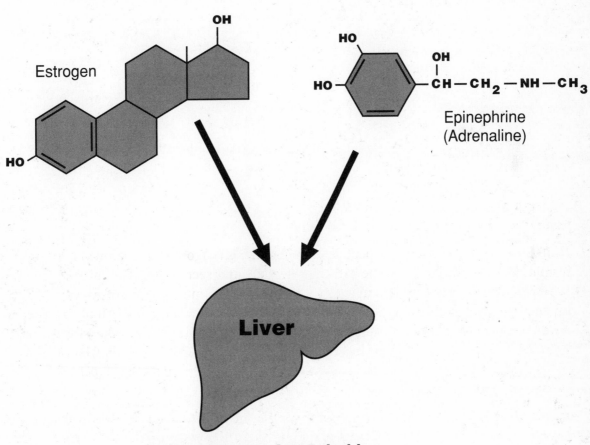

Estrogen

Epinephrine
(Adrenaline)

Liver

**Hormones are degraded by
enzymes in the liver**

Part II : Self-Testing Exercises

Unlabeled illustrations from Part I

MAJOR ENDOCRINE GLANDS

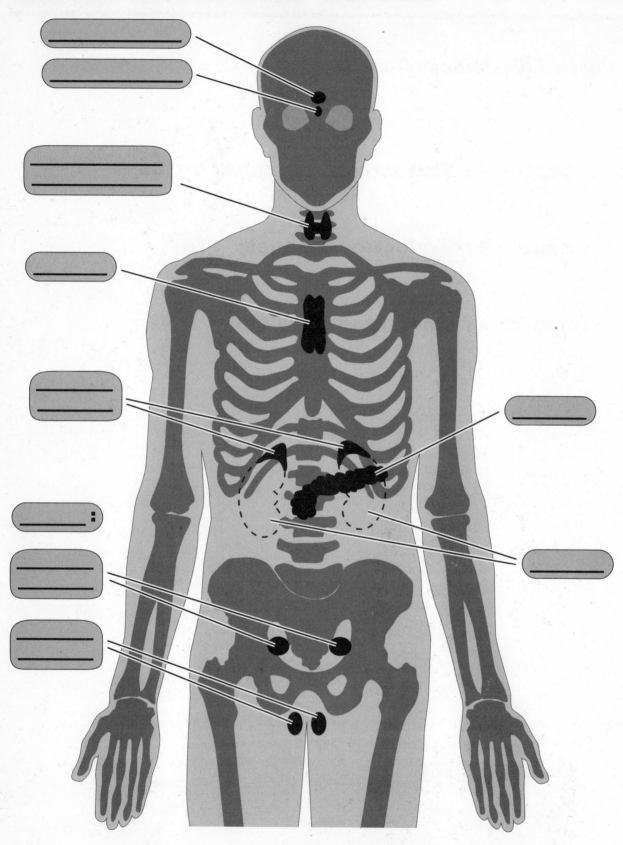

GLANDS

_____ Glands

_____ gland cells secrete their products into ducts that empty at the skin surface or into the lumen of a hollow organ.

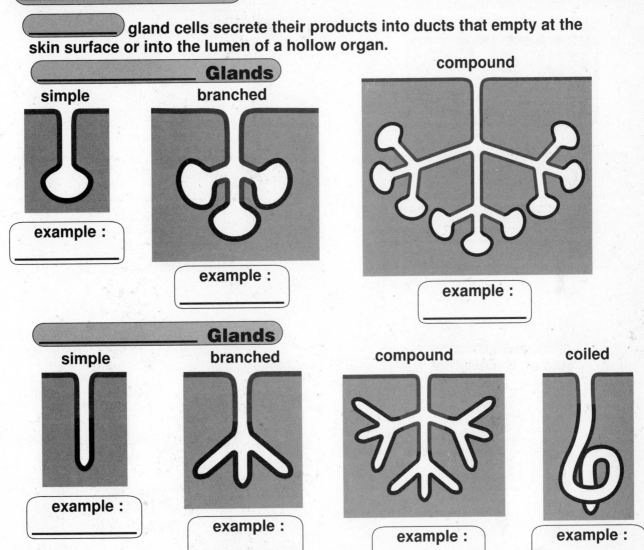

_____ Glands

simple

example :
_____

branched

example :
_____

compound

example :
_____

_____ Glands

simple

example :
_____

branched

example :
_____

compound

example :
_____

coiled

example :
_____

_____ Glands

_____ gland cells secrete hormones into nearby capillaries.

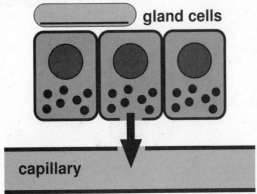

_____ gland cells

capillary

CHEMICAL MESSENGERS

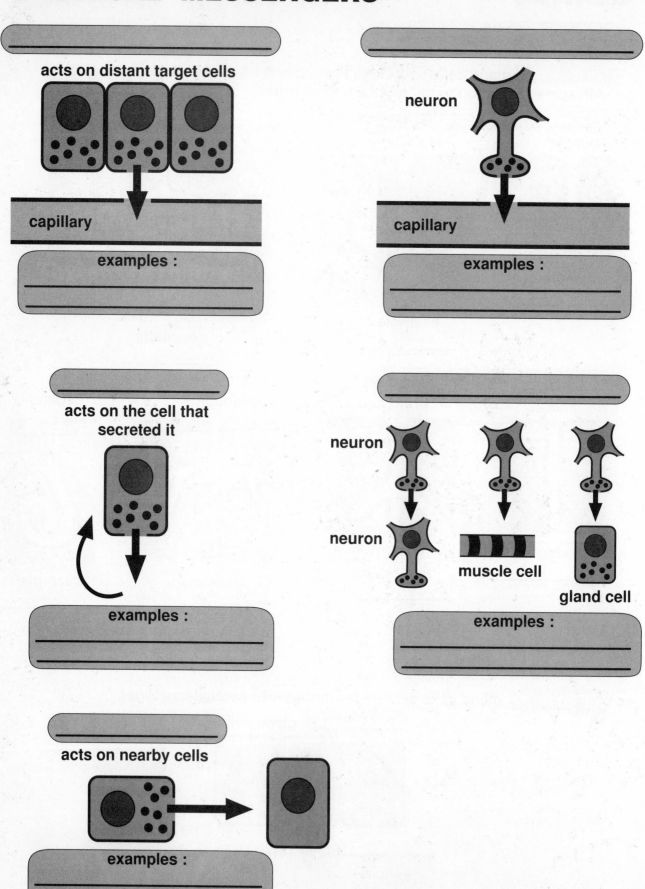

acts on distant target cells

capillary

examples :

_____
_____

neuron

capillary

examples :

_____
_____

acts on the cell that
secreted it

examples :

_____
_____

neuron

neuron

muscle cell

gland cell

examples :

_____
_____

acts on nearby cells

examples :

_____
_____

70

HORMONE FUNCTIONS

Functions	Some Hormones Involved
(_____)	Thyroxine, Epinephrine, hGH, GHIH, Insulin, Glucagon
(_____)	Gastrin, Secretin, CCK, GHIH, Gastric Inhibitory Peptide
(_____)	GnRH, FSH, LH, Prolactin, Progesterone, Estrogen, Inhibin, Oxytocin, Relaxin, Testosterone, Human Chorionic Gonadotropin, Human Chorionic Somatomammotropin
(_____)	Epinephrine, Aldosterone, Antidiuretic Hormone, Angiotensin II, Histamine, Atrial Natriuretic Peptide
(_____)	Calcitonin, Calcitriol, Parathyroid Hormone
(_____)	Insulin, Glucagon, Epinephrine, GHIH
(_____)	Aldosterone
(_____)	Erythropoietin (red blood cells), Thymosin (white blood cells)
(_____)	Human Growth Hormone, Thyroid Hormones, Insulin, Testosterone, Estrogens
(_____)	Interferons, Interleukins, Tumor Necrosis Factor, Lymphotoxin, Perforin, Thymosin
(_____)	Cortisol, Epinephrine, Aldosterone, Antidiuretic Hormone, Growth Hormone, Glucagon

INTERFERONS

Virus-infected macrophages release interferons (IFNs). The interferons diffuse to neighboring cells and bind to surface receptors. This induces the uninfected cells to synthesize antiviral proteins that interfere with or inhibit viral replication.

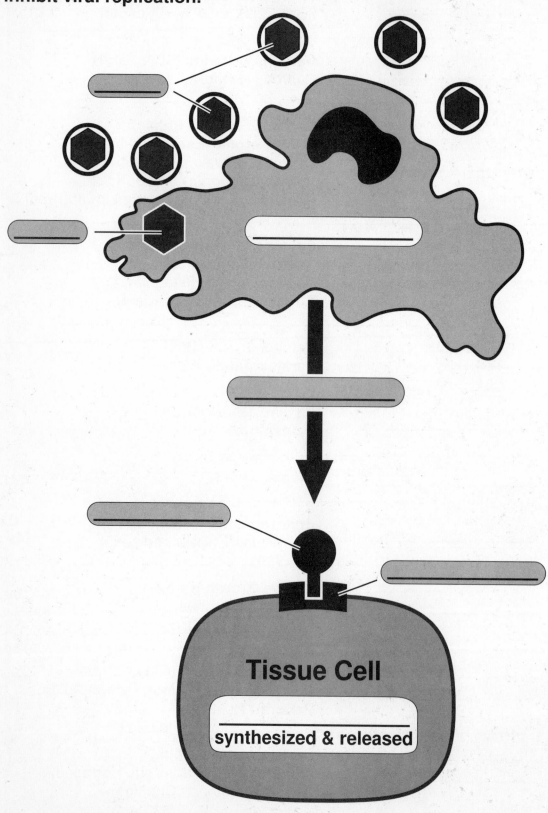

Tissue Cell

_____
synthesized & released

HORMONE CLASSIFICATION :

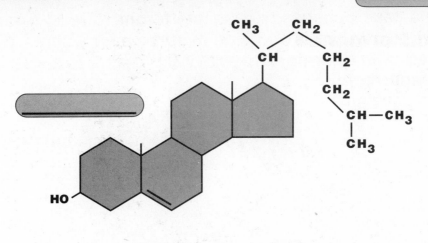

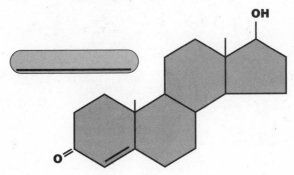

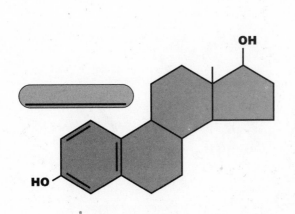

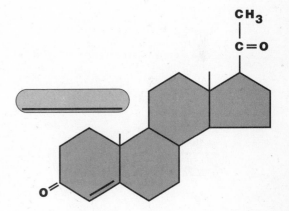

73

HORMONE CLASSIFICATION :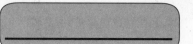

Thyroid Hormones

(___)

HO ─⬡─ O ─⬡─ CH₂ ─ CH ─ COOH
                              |
                             NH₂

(___)

HO ─⬡─ O ─⬡─ CH₂ ─ CH ─ COOH
                              |
                             NH₂

Catecholamines

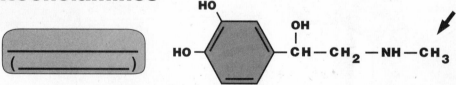

(_____)

HO ─⬡─ CH ─ CH₂ ─ NH ─ CH₃
HO |
        OH

(_____)

HO ─⬡─ CH ─ CH₂ ─ NH₂
HO |
        OH

74

HORMONE CLASSIFICATION : _____

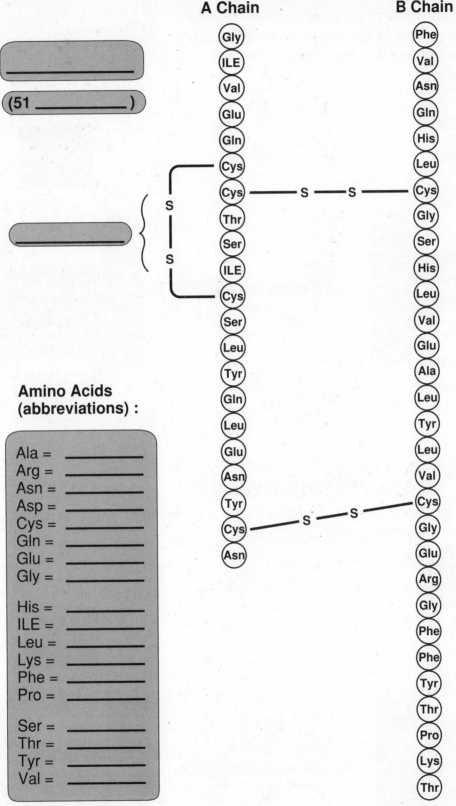

A Chain

Gly
ILE
Val
Glu
Gln
Cys
Cys
Thr
Ser
ILE
Cys
Ser
Leu
Tyr
Gln
Leu
Glu
Asn
Tyr
Cys
Asn

B Chain

Phe
Val
Asn
Gln
His
Leu
Cys
Gly
Ser
His
Leu
Val
Glu
Ala
Leu
Tyr
Leu
Val
Cys
Gly
Glu
Arg
Gly
Phe
Phe
Tyr
Thr
Pro
Lys
Thr

_____

(51 _____)

_____

Amino Acids (abbreviations) :

Ala = _____
Arg = _____
Asn = _____
Asp = _____
Cys = _____
Gln = _____
Glu = _____
Gly = _____

His = _____
ILE = _____
Leu = _____
Lys = _____
Phe = _____
Pro = _____

Ser = _____
Thr = _____
Tyr = _____
Val = _____

RECEPTOR MODULATION

_____ Modulation

A modulator molecule binds to one binding site (the _____ site) of a receptor; this alters the shape of a second binding site (the _____ site).

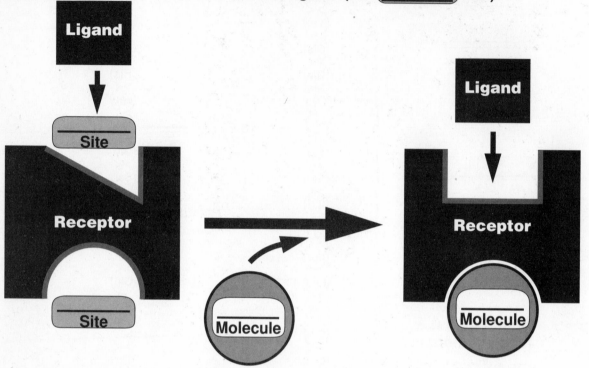

_____ Modulation

A _____ catalyzes the binding of a phosphate group with a receptor; this alters the shape of the _____ site.

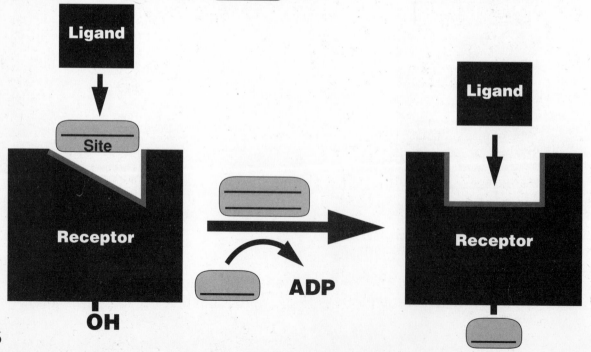

HORMONE ACTION

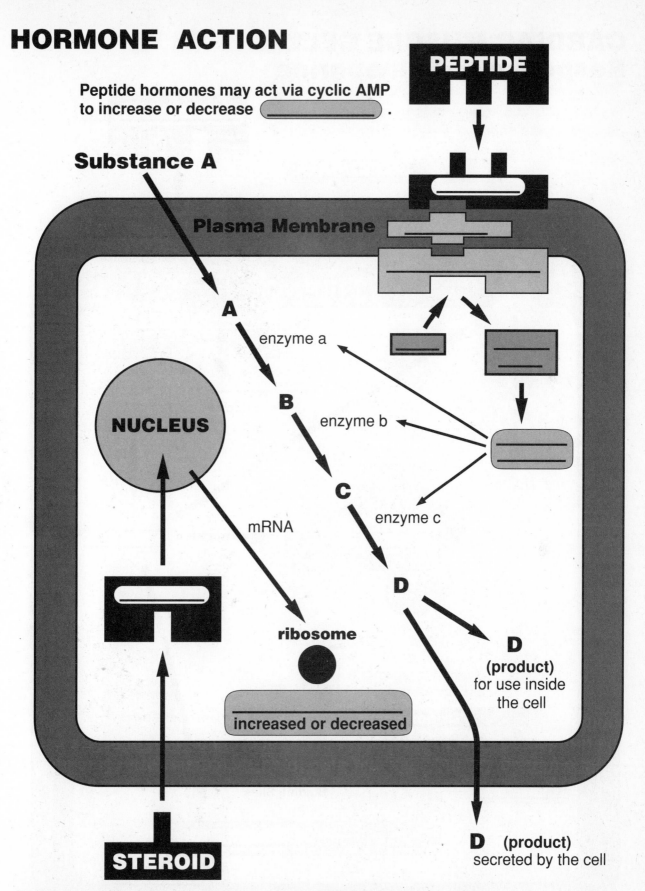

Peptide hormones may act via cyclic AMP to increase or decrease _____ .

PEPTIDE

Substance A

Plasma Membrane

A

enzyme a

B

NUCLEUS

enzyme b

C

mRNA

enzyme c

D

ribosome

D (product) for use inside the cell

increased or decreased

STEROID

D (product) secreted by the cell

Some hormones may "turn on" or "turn off" genes in the nucleus, causing an increase or decrease in the _____ of specific proteins (enzymes).

CARDIAC MUSCLE CELL
Response to Epinephrine

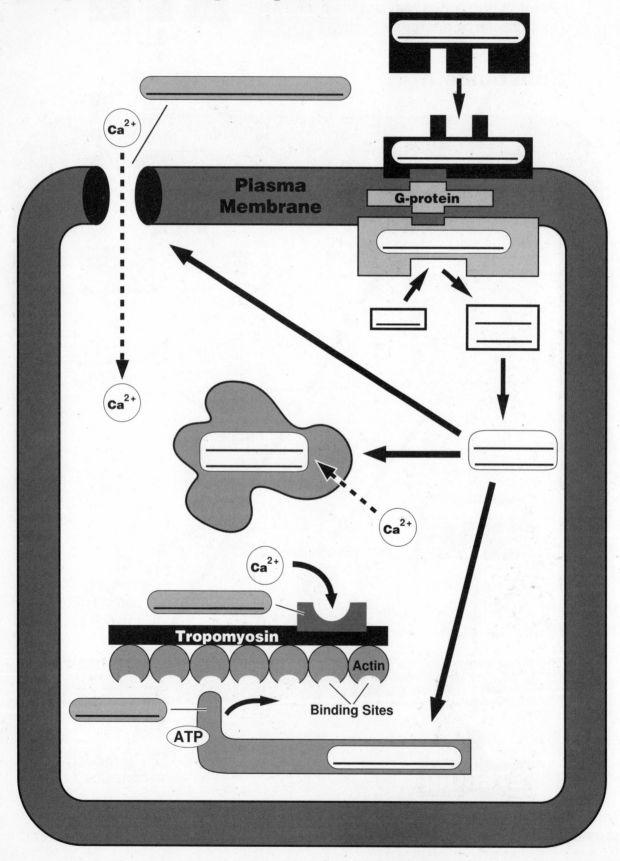

HYPOTHALAMUS

Neurons in the hypothalamus secrete neurohormones.

9 tropic hormones travel to the anterior pituitary via portal vessels.
(_____ and _____) travel down long axons
and are released into the general circulation in the posterior pituitary.

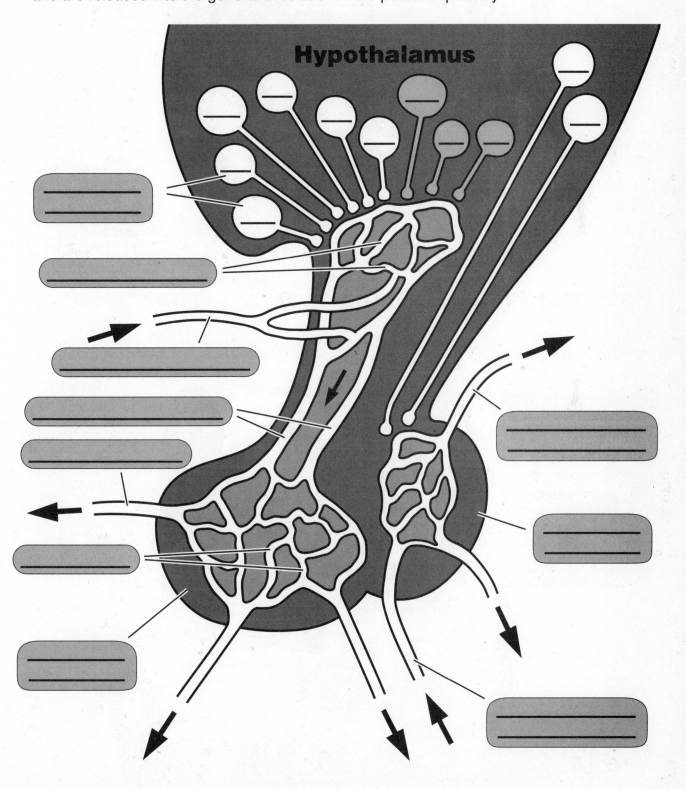

PITUITARY GLAND

Location

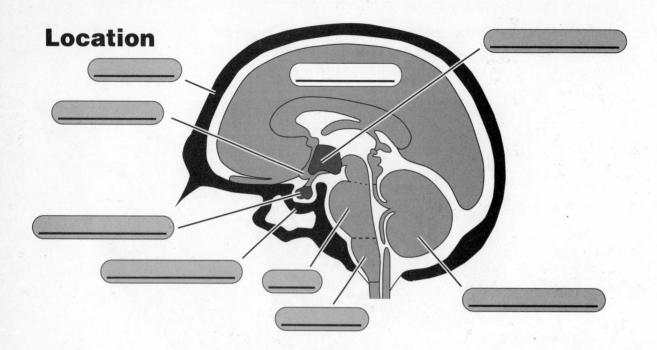

Posterior Pituitary Gland

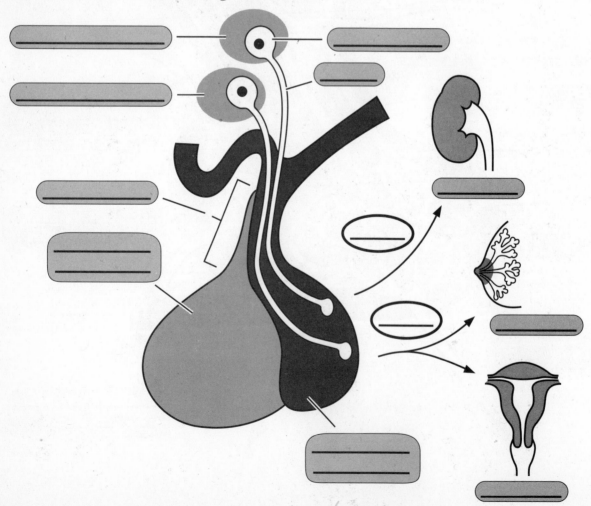

ANTERIOR PITUITARY GLAND

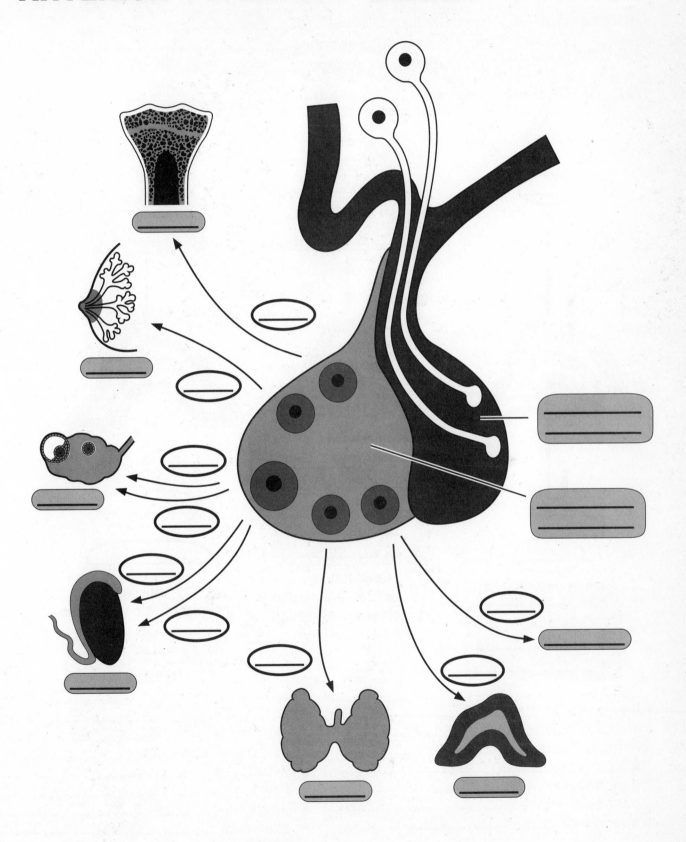

ADRENAL GLANDS

Adrenal Cortex : zona fasciculata secretes _____
zona glomerulosa secretes _____
zona reticularis secretes _____

Adrenal Medulla : secretes _____ and _____

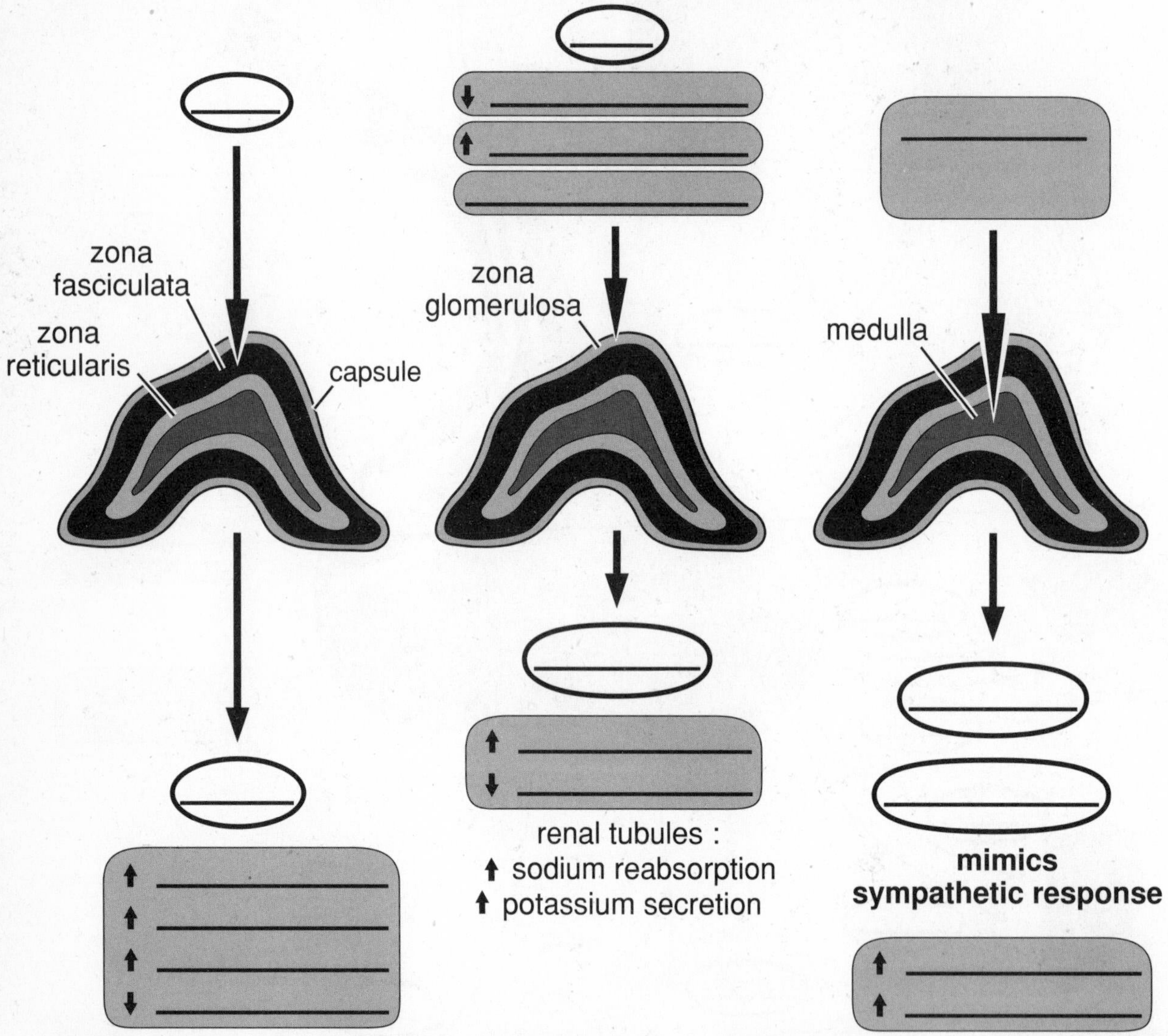

zona
fasciculata

zona
reticularis

capsule

zona
glomerulosa

medulla

renal tubules :
↑ sodium reabsorption
↑ potassium secretion

**mimics
sympathetic response**

body cells : _____
skeletal muscle : _____
adipose tissue : _____
liver : _____
lymphocytes : _____
connective tissue : _____
arterioles : _____

body cells : _____
skeletal muscle : _____
adipose tissue : _____
liver : _____
heart : _____
lungs : _____
eyes : _____
anterior pituitary : _____
blood plasma : _____
arterioles : _____

THYROID and PARATHYROID GLANDS

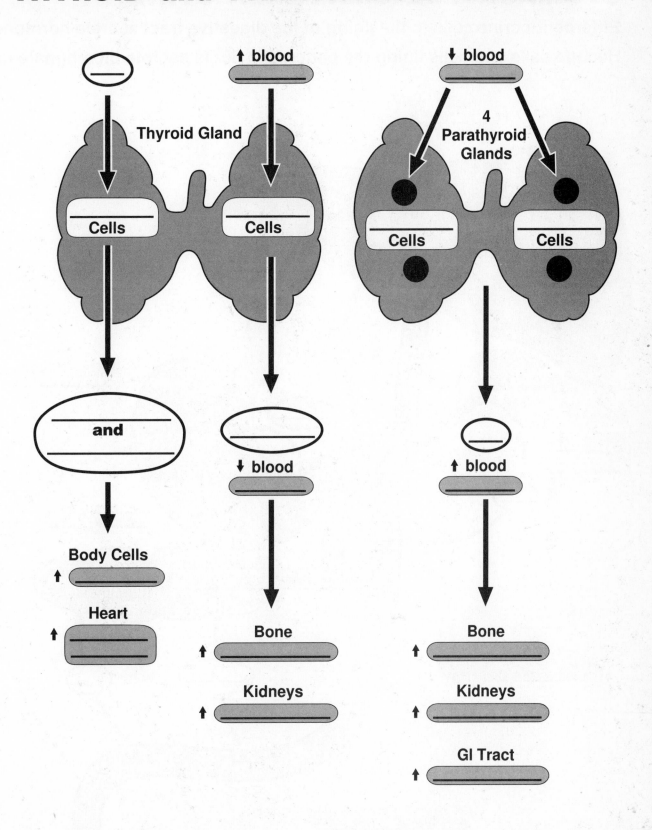

Thyroid Gland

Cells

Cells

↑ blood

↓ blood

4
Parathyroid
Glands

Cells

Cells

and

↓ blood

↑ blood

Body Cells

↑

Heart

↑

Bone

↑

Kidneys

↑

Bone

↑

Kidneys

↑

GI Tract

↑

STOMACH and SMALL INTESTINE

Enteroendocrine cells in the lining of the digestive tract secrete hormones.
Hepatic cells and cells lining the pancreatic ducts secrete bicarbonate ions.

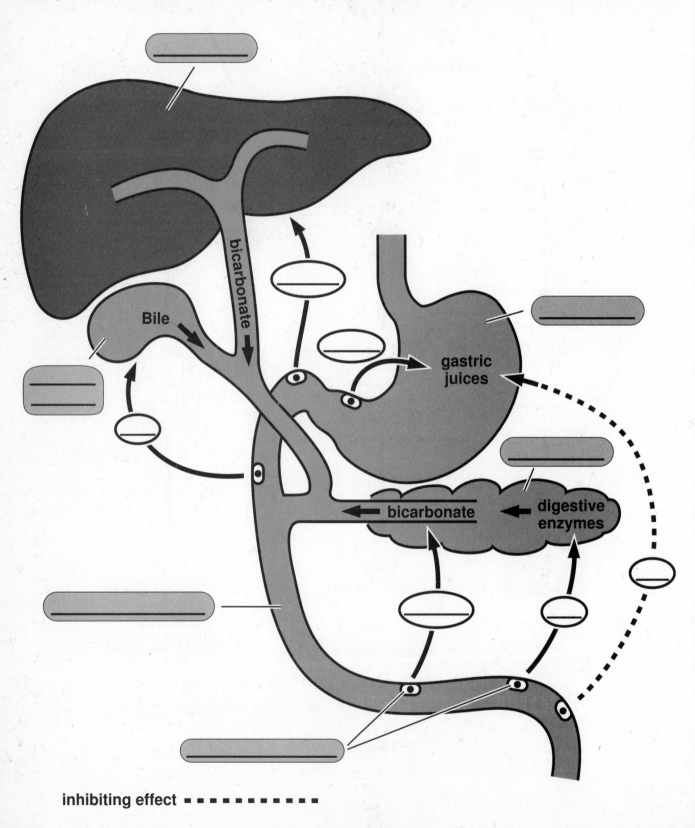

inhibiting effect ▪ ▪ ▪ ▪ ▪ ▪ ▪ ▪ ▪

PANCREATIC ISLETS
Alpha and Beta Cell secretions (D-cells and F-cells not illustrated)

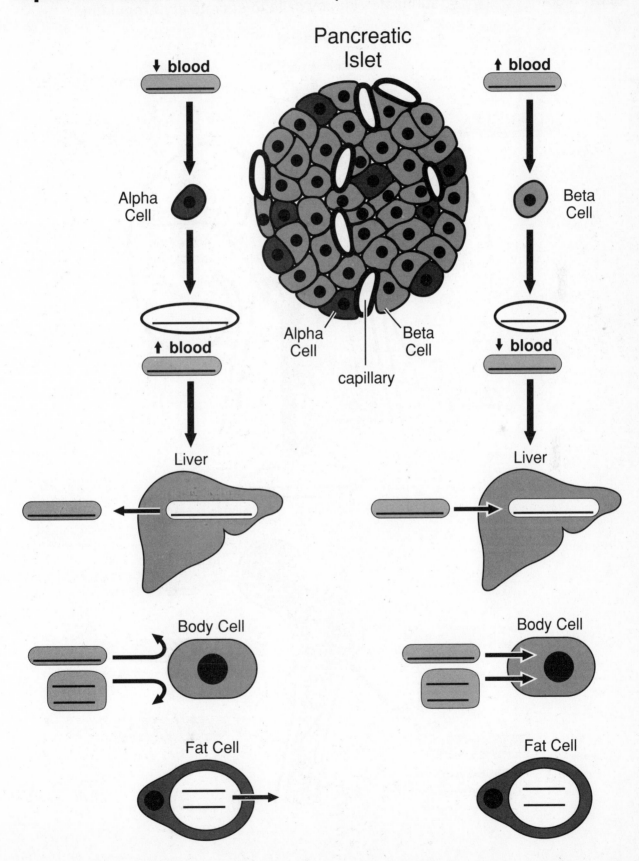

KIDNEYS

Low blood _____ stimulates kidney cells to secrete erythropoietin.

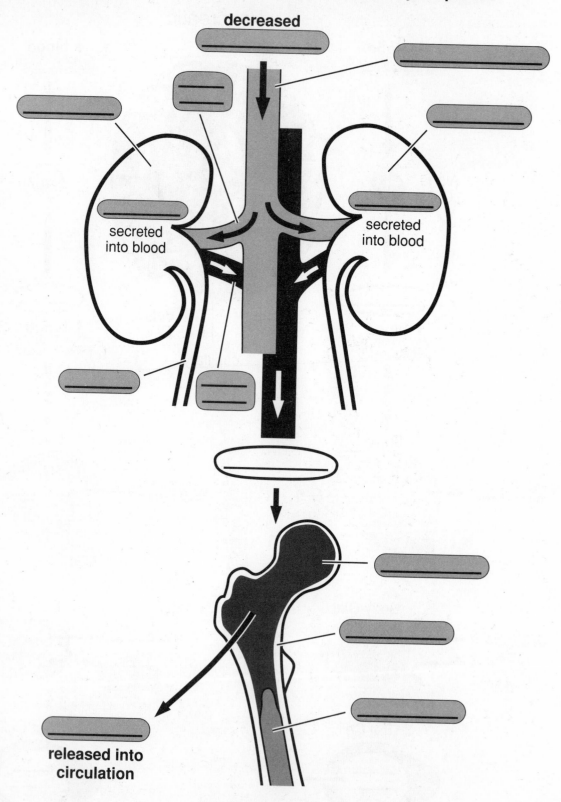

decreased

secreted
into blood

secreted
into blood

released into
circulation

TESTES

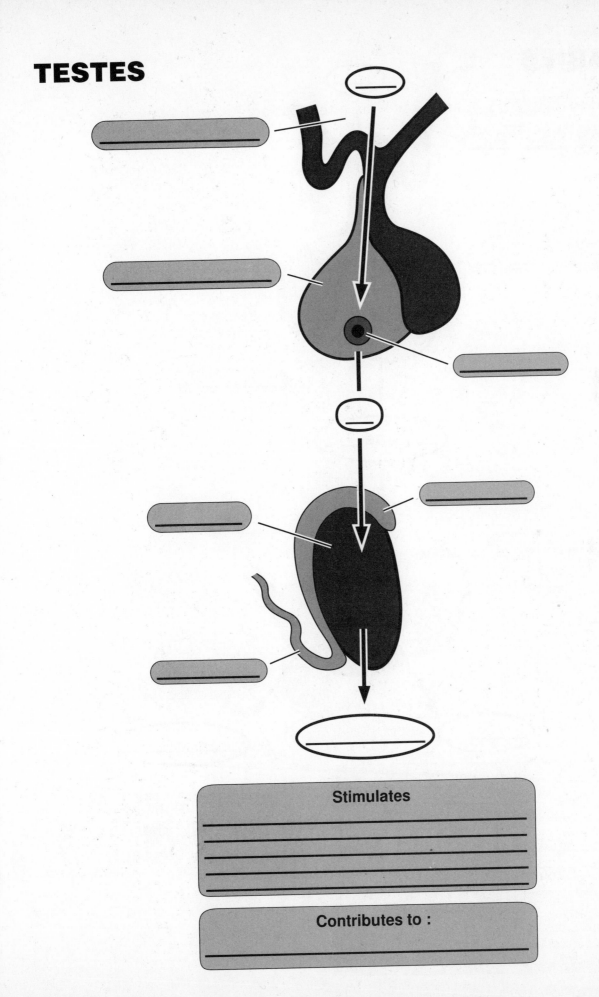

Stimulates

_____

_____

_____

_____

_____

Contributes to :

_____

_____

OVARIES

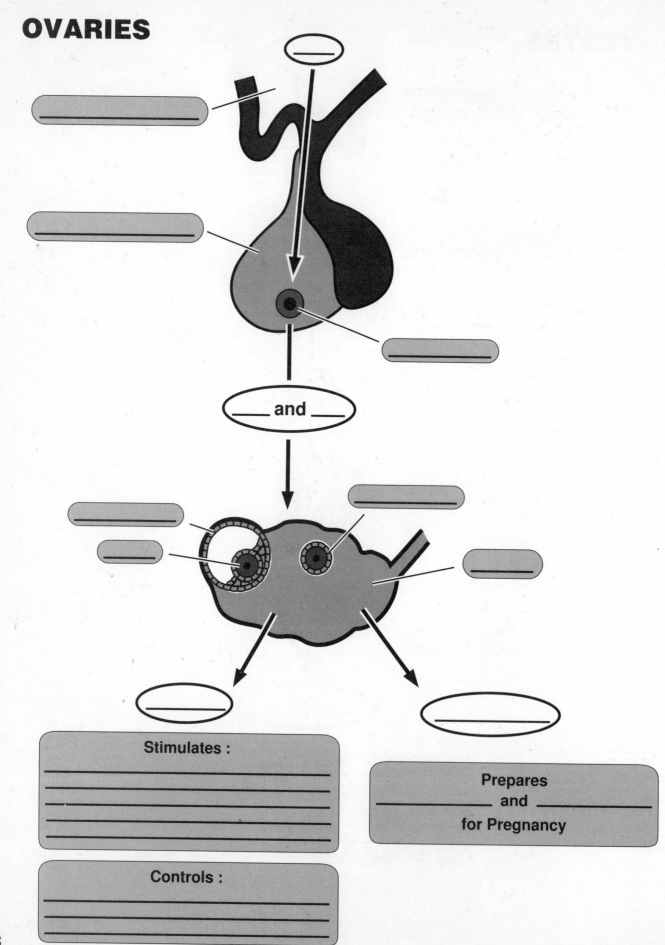

Stimulates :
_____
_____
_____
_____
_____

Controls :
_____
_____
_____

Prepares
_____ and _____
for Pregnancy

PINEAL GLAND, HEART, and LIVER

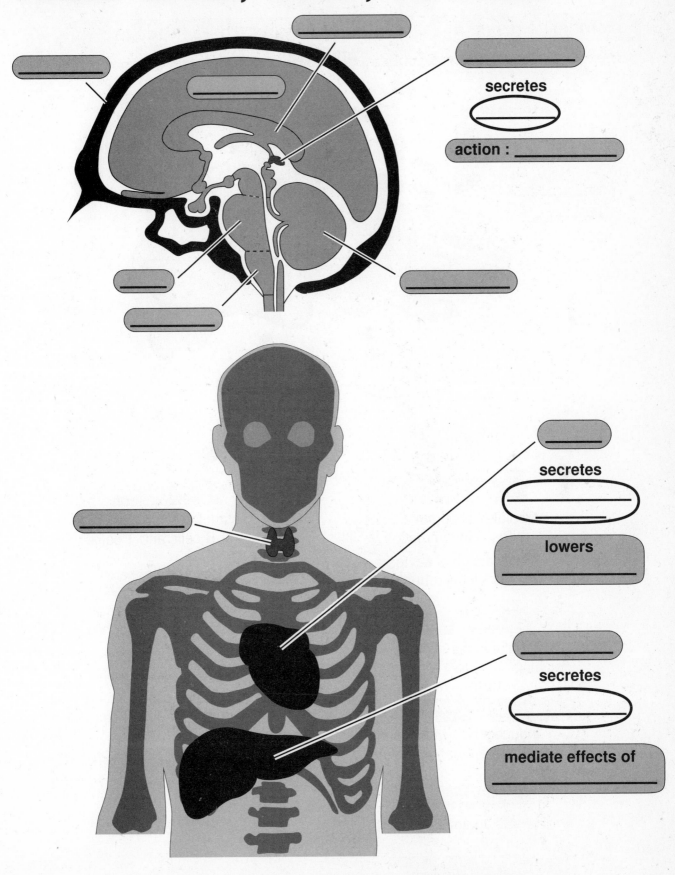

secretes
action : _____

secretes
_____

lowers
_____

secretes
_____

mediate effects of
_____

MACROPHAGES

Microbes ingested by macrophages stimulate the release of
_____ and _____

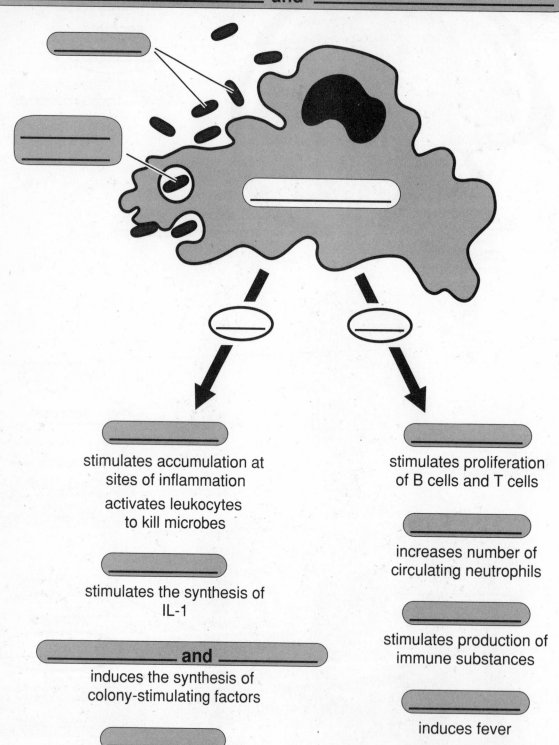

_____

_____

_____

_____

_____
stimulates accumulation at
sites of inflammation

activates leukocytes
to kill microbes

_____
stimulates the synthesis of
IL-1

_____ and _____
induces the synthesis of
colony-stimulating factors

_____
exerts an antiviral effect

_____
induces fever

_____
stimulates proliferation
of B cells and T cells

_____
increases number of
circulating neutrophils

_____
stimulates production of
immune substances

_____
induces fever

CONTROL OF HORMONE SECRETION
Negative Feedback

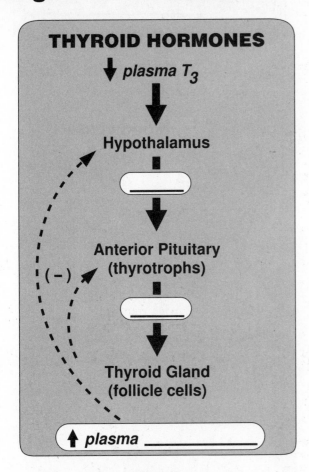

THYROID HORMONES

↓ *plasma T₃*

Hypothalamus

Anterior Pituitary
(thyrotrophs)

(–)

Thyroid Gland
(follicle cells)

↑ *plasma* _____

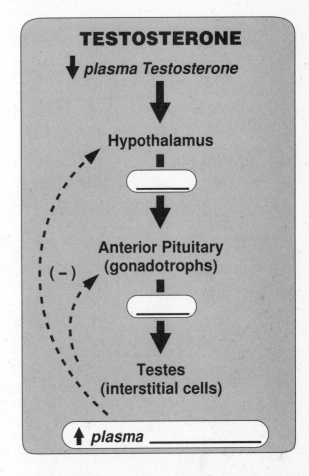

TESTOSTERONE

↓ *plasma Testosterone*

Hypothalamus

Anterior Pituitary
(gonadotrophs)

(–)

Testes
(interstitial cells)

↑ *plasma* _____

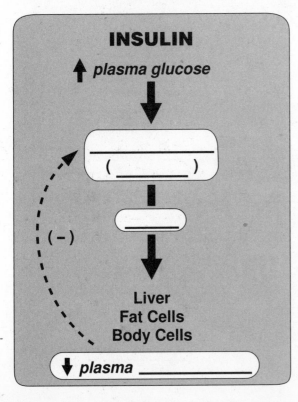

INSULIN

↑ *plasma glucose*

(_____)

(–)

Liver
Fat Cells
Body Cells

↓ *plasma* _____

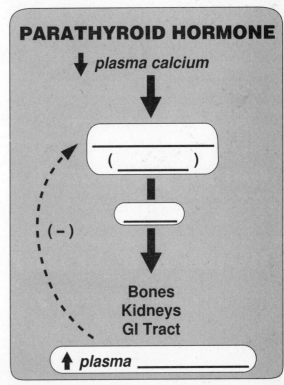

PARATHYROID HORMONE

↓ *plasma calcium*

(_____)

(–)

Bones
Kidneys
GI Tract

↑ *plasma* _____

THYROID HORMONE
Synthesis and Action

key :

TGB = _____

TSH = _____

TBG = _____

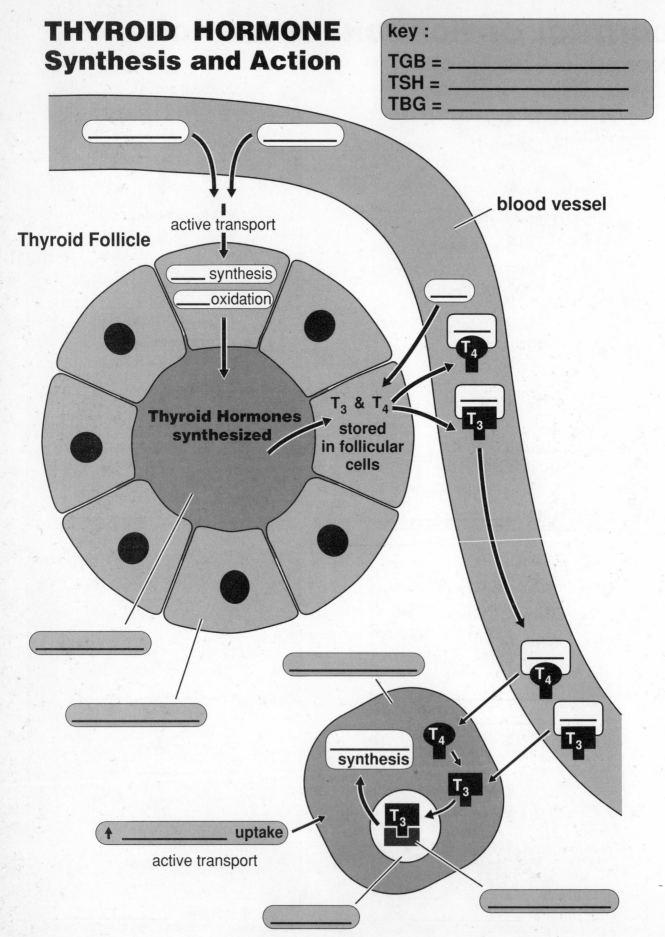

blood vessel

active transport

Thyroid Follicle

_____ synthesis

_____ oxidation

Thyroid Hormones synthesized

T_3 & T_4 stored in follicular cells

T_4

T_3

synthesis

T_4

T_3

T_3

↑ _____ uptake

active transport

ANTAGONISTIC HORMONES

_____ : stimulates the conversion of glucose to glycogen (uptake of glucose).

_____ : stimulates the conversion of glycogen to glucose (release of glucose).

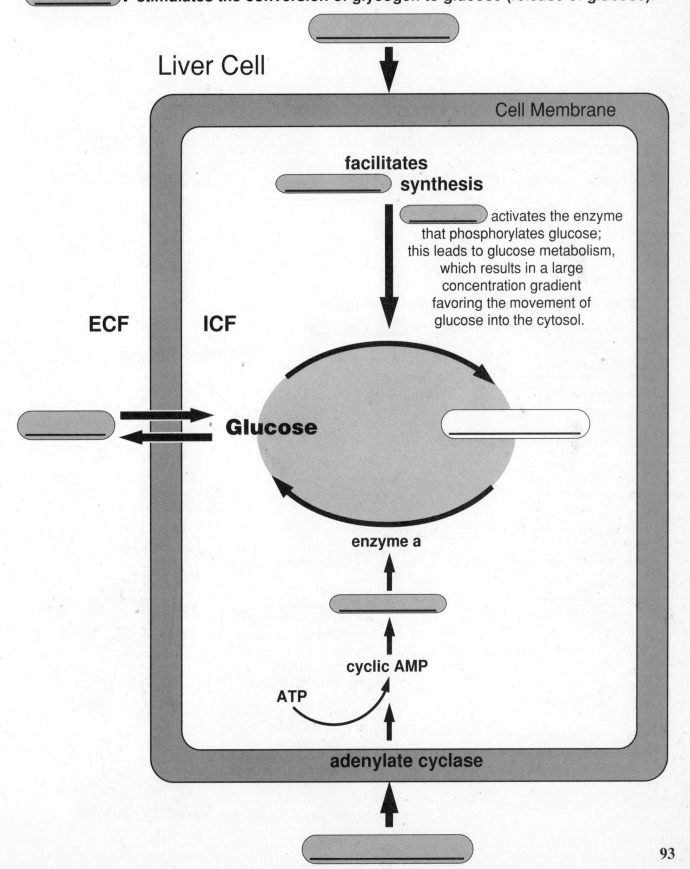

Liver Cell

Cell Membrane

facilitates
_____ synthesis

_____ activates the enzyme that phosphorylates glucose; this leads to glucose metabolism, which results in a large concentration gradient favoring the movement of glucose into the cytosol.

ECF   ICF

Glucose

_____

enzyme a

_____

cyclic AMP

ATP

adenylate cyclase

STRESS RESPONSE (General Adaptation Syndrome)

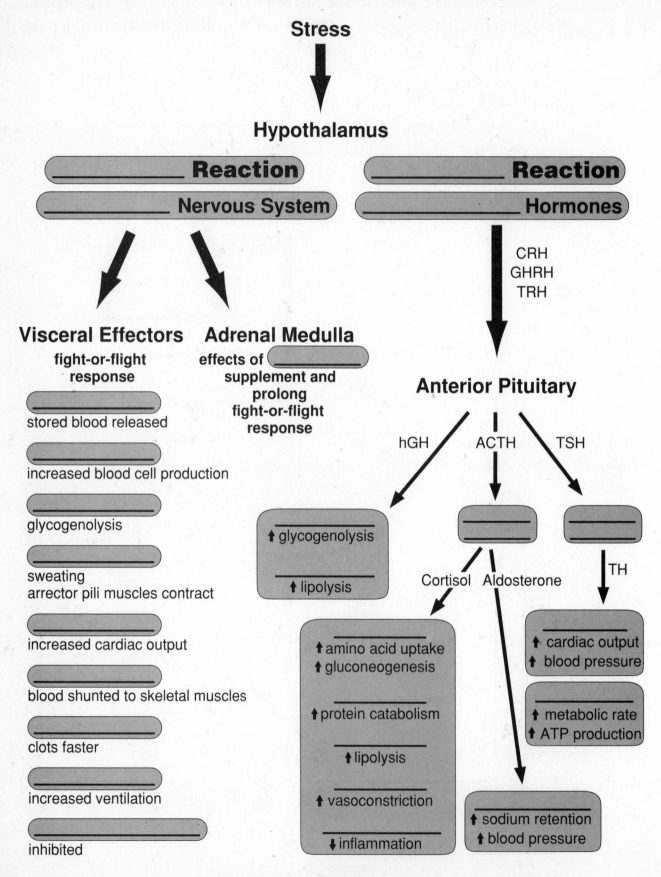

Stress

Hypothalamus

_____ **Reaction**

_____ **Nervous System**

_____ **Reaction**

_____ **Hormones**

CRH
GHRH
TRH

Visceral Effectors

fight-or-flight response

stored blood released

increased blood cell production

glycogenolysis

sweating
arrector pili muscles contract

increased cardiac output

blood shunted to skeletal muscles

clots faster

increased ventilation

inhibited

Adrenal Medulla

effects of _____ supplement and prolong fight-or-flight response

Anterior Pituitary

hGH   ACTH   TSH

_____
↑glycogenolysis
_____
↑lipolysis

Cortisol   Aldosterone

_____
↑amino acid uptake
↑gluconeogenesis
_____
↑protein catabolism
_____
↑lipolysis
_____
↑vasoconstriction
_____
↓inflammation

TH

↑cardiac output
↑blood pressure

↑metabolic rate
↑ATP production

↑sodium retention
↑blood pressure

CALCIUM BALANCE
Calcium homeostasis is regulated by
Parathyroid Hormone (PTH), Calcitriol, and Calcitonin

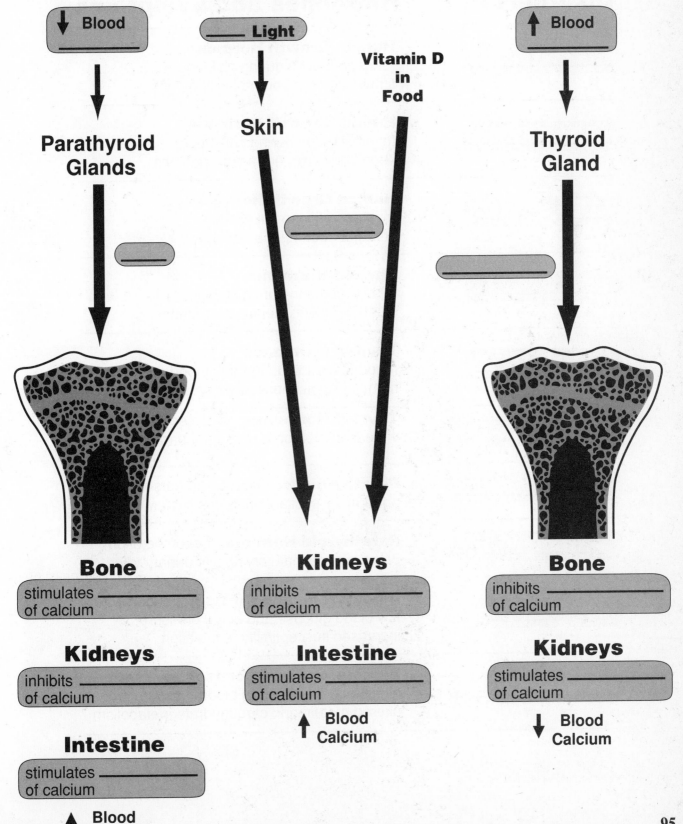

↓ Blood
_____

_____ Light

Vitamin D
in
Food

↑ Blood
_____

Parathyroid
Glands

Skin

Thyroid
Gland

Bone

stimulates _____
of calcium

Kidneys

inhibits _____
of calcium

Bone

inhibits _____
of calcium

Kidneys

inhibits _____
of calcium

Intestine

stimulates _____
of calcium

Kidneys

stimulates _____
of calcium

↑ Blood
Calcium

↓ Blood
Calcium

Intestine

stimulates _____
of calcium

↑ Blood
Calcium

HORMONE DISORDERS

Disorders	Hormones and Symptoms
_____	**Human Growth Hormone** (undersecretion during childhood) small body size; normal proportions
_____	**Human Growth Hormone** (oversecretion during childhood) large body size; normal proportions
_____	**Human Growth Hormone** (oversecretion in adulthood) enlarged feet, hands, and jaw
_____	**Thyroid Hormones** (undersecretion during childhood) stunted growth; mental retardation
_____	**Thyroid Hormones** (undersecretion during adulthood) mental sluggishness; dry skin; fatigue
_____	**Thyroid Hormones** (oversecretion) increased metabolic rate and heart rate
_____	**Parathyroid Hormone** (undersecretion) abnormally excitable nervous system
_____	**Parathyroid Hormone** (oversecretion) calcium phosphate crystals in urinary tract
_____	**Aldosterone and Cortisol** (undersecretion) low blood glucose and blood pressure; increased susceptibility to infection
_____	**Aldosterone and Cortisol** (oversecretion) high blood glucose and blood pressure; altered protein and carbohydrate metabolism

DIABETES MELLITUS

_____ Deficiency (glucagon excess)

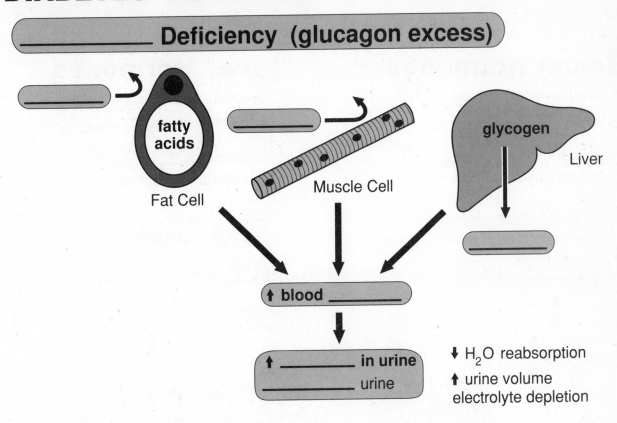

↓ H₂O reabsorption

↑ urine volume electrolyte depletion

Metabolism of Noncarbohydrates

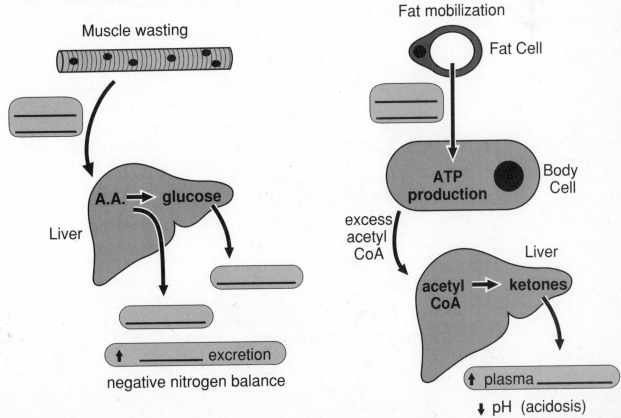

HORMONE ELIMINATION

Bound Hormones

circulate in the blood
bound to (_____)

difficult to (_____)
remain active for hours

(_____)

(_____)

"Free" Hormones

circulate "free" in the plasma
(unbound to (_____))

easy to (_____)
inactivated in minutes

(_____)

(_____)

(_____)

Estrogen

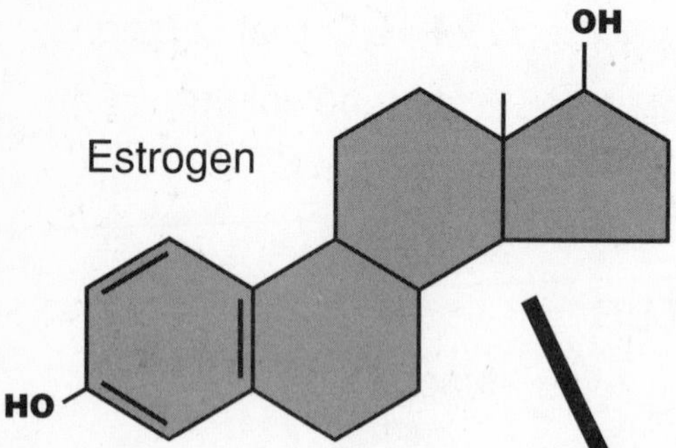

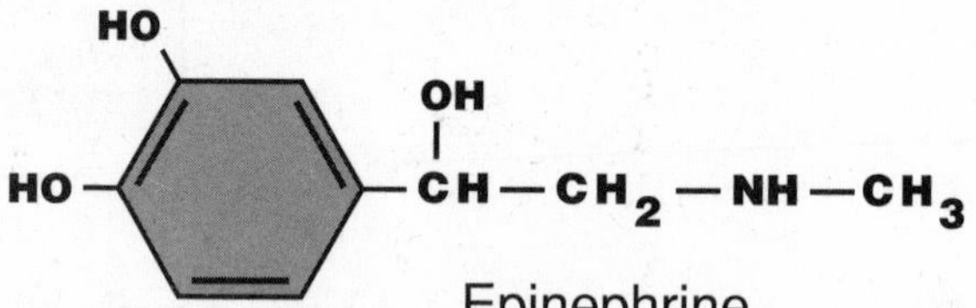

Epinephrine
(Adrenaline)

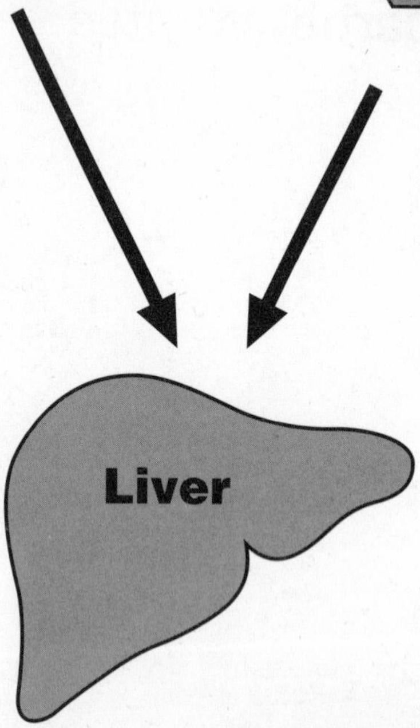

Liver

Hormones are (_____)
by enzymes in the liver

Part III : Terminology

Pronunciation Guide

acetyl CoA   AS - e - til kō - Ā
acetyl coenzyme A   AS - e - til kō - EN - zīm - Ā
acidosis   as - i - DŌ - sis
acinar   AS - i - nar
acini   AS - i - nē
acromegaly   ak′ - rō - MEG - a - lē
adenohypophysis   ad′ - e - nō - hī - POF - i - sis
adenylate cyclase   a - DEN - i - lāt SĪ - klās
adrenal   a - DRĒ - nal
adrenaline   a - DREN - a - lin
adrenocorticotropic   ad - rē′ - nō - kor′ - ti - kō - TRŌ - pik
adrenocorticotropin   ad - rē′ - nō - kor′ - ti - kō - TRŌ - pin
aldosterone   al - DA - ster - ōn
allosteric   al′ - ō - STER - ik
alpha   AL - fa
amine   a - MĒN
anabolism   a - NAB - ō - lizm
androgen   AN - drō - jen
angiotensin   an′ - jē - ō - TEN - sin
angiotensinogen   an′ - jē - ō - TEN - sin - ō - jen
antagonistic   an - tag - ō - NIST - ik
anterior   an - TĒR - ē - or
antidiuretic   an′ - ti - dī - yoo - RET - ik
apocrine   AP - ō - krin
arachidonic   a - ra - ki - DON - ik
arteriole   ar - TĒ - rē - ōl
atrial   Ā - trē - al
autocrine   AW - tō - krin
basal   BĀ - sal
beta   BĀ - ta
bile   BĪL
biogenic amine   bī - ō - JEN - ik a - MĒN
calcitonin   kal - si - TŌ - nin

calcitriol   kal - si - TRĪ - ol
calorigenic   ka - lor′ - i - JEN - ik
catabolism   ka - TAB - ō - lizm
catecholamine   kat′ - e - KOL - a - mēn
cholecalciferol   kō′ - lē - kal - SIF - er - ōl
cholecystokinin   kō′ - lē - sis′ - tō - KĪ - nin
cholesterol   kō - LES - te - rol
chorionic   kō′ - rē - ON - ik
chromaffin   krō - MAF - in
colloid   KOL - oyd
corpus luteum   KOR - pus LOO - tē - um
corticosterone   kor′ - ti - KOS - ter - ōn
corticotroph   KOR - ti - kō - trōf
corticotropin   kor′ - ti - kō - TRŌ - pin
cortisol   KOR - ti - sol
cortisone   KOR - ti - sōn
cretinism   KRĒ - tin - izm
cyclic   SĪ - klik
cytokine   SĪ - tō - kīn
cytosol   SĪ - tō - sol
diabetes   dī - a - BĒ - tēz
diencephalon   dī′ - en - SEF - a - lon
diffusion   dif - YOO - zhun
dihydrotestosterone   dī - hī′ - drō - tes - TOS - ter - ōn
dihydroxy   dī - hī - DROK - sē
diuresis   dī′ - yoo - RĒ - sis
duodenum   doo′ - ō - DĒ - num
eicosanoid   ī - KŌ - sa - noyd
electrolyte   ē - LEK - trō - līt
endocrine   EN - dō - krin
endocrinology   en′ - dō - kri - NOL - ō - jē
enzyme   En - zīm
epinephrine   ep - ē - NEF - rin

epiphysis cerebri ē-PIF-i-sis se-RĒ-brē
erythropoiesis e-rith′-rō-poy-Ē-sis
erythropoietin e-rith′-rō-POY-ē-tin
estrogens ES-trō-jens
exocrine EK-sō-krin
exocytosis ex′-ō-sī-TŌ-sis
fibroblast FĪ-brō-blast
follicle Fol-i-kul
follicular fō-LIK-yoo-lar
gastrin GAS-trin
gene JĒN
giantism JĪ-an-tizm
globulin GLOB-yoo-lin
glucagon GLOO-ka-gon
glucocorticoids gloo′-kō-KOR-ti-koyds
glucogenesis gloo′-kō-JEN-e-sis
gluconeogenesis gloo′-kō-nē′-ō-JEN-e-sis
glycogenesis glī′-kō-JEN-e-sis
glycogenolysis glī′-kō-je-NOL-i-sis
glycosuria glī′-kō-SOO-rē-a
gonad GŌ-nad
gonadocorticoids gō′-na-dō-KOR-ti-koyds
gonadotroph gō-NAD-ō-trōf
gonadotropin gō′-nad-ō-TRŌ-pin
hematopoietic hem′-a-tō-poy-ET-ik
histamine HISS-ta-mēn
histadine HISS-ti-dēn
holocrine HŌL-ō-krin
homeostasis hō′-mē-ō-STĀ-sis
hormone HOR-mōn
hydrochloric hī′-drō-KLOR-ik
hydrocortisone hī′-drō-KOR-ti-sōn
hypercalcemia hī′-per-kal-SĒ-mē-a
hyperglycemia hī′-per-glī-SĒ-mē-a
hypersecretion hī′-per-se-KRĒ-shun
hypertension hī′-per-TEN-shun
hypertonic hī′-per-TON-ik
hypocalcemia hī′-pō-kal-SĒ-mē-a
hypoglycemia hī′-pō-glī-SĒ-mē-a
hypokalemia hī′-pō-kā-LĒ-mē-a
hyponatremia hī′-pō-na-TRĒ-mē-a
hypophyseal hī′-pō-FIZ-ē-al
hypophysiotropic hī′-pō-fiz-ē-ō-TRŌ-pik
hypophysis hī-POF-i-sis
hyposecretion hī′-pō-se-KRĒ-shun
hypothalamic hī′-pō-thal-AM-ik
hypothalamus hī′-pō-THAL-a-mus
hypotonic hī′-pō-TON-ik
infundibulum in-fun-DIB-yoo-lum
inhibin in-HIB-in
insipidus in-SIP-i-dus
insulin IN-su-lin
interferon in′-ter-FĒR-on
interleukin in′-ter-LOO-kin

interstitial in′-ter-STISH-al
ion Ī-on
islet Ī-lit
isthmus IS-mus
juxtaglomerular juks-ta-glō-MER-yoo-lar
ketone KĒ-tōn
ketosis kē-TŌ-sis
kinase KĪ-nās
lactation lak-TĀ-shun
lactogenic lak′-tō-JEN-ik
lactotroph LAK-tō-trōf
Langerhans LAHNG-er-hanz
lateral LAT-er-al
leukotriene loo′-kō-TRĪ-ēn
Leydig LĪ-dig
ligand LĪ-gand
lipid LI-pid
lipogenesis li-pō-GEN-e-sis
lipolysis li-POL-i-sis
luteinizing LOO-tē-in-īz-ing
lymphocyte LIM-fō-sīt
lymphokine LIM-fō-kīn
melanocyte MEL-a-nō-sīt
melatonin mel-a-TŌN-in
mellitus MEL-i-tus
merocrine MER-ō-krin
mineralocorticoid min′-er-al-ō-KOR-ti-koyd
monocyte MON-ō-sīt
monokine MON-ō-kīn
myxedema mix-e-DĒ-ma
natriuretic nā′-trē-yoo-RET-ik
neuroendocrine noo′-rō-EN-dō-krin
neurohypophysis noo′-rō-hī-POF-i-sis
neurosecretory noo′-rō-SĒK-re-tō-rē
noradrenaline nor′-a-DREN-a-lin
norepinephrine nor′-ep-ē-NEF-rin
osmoreceptor oz′-mō-re-SEP-tor
osmotic diuresis oz-MOT-ik dī-yoo-RĒ-sis
ovary Ō-var-ē
oxyphil OK-sē-fil
oxytocin ok′-sē-TŌ-sin
pancreas PAN-krē-as
pancreatic pan′-krē-AT-ik
paracrine PAR-a-krin
parafollicular par′-a-fō-LIK-yoo-lar
parathormone par′-a-THOR-mōn
parathyroid par′-a-THĪ-royd
pars intermedia PARZ in-ter-MĒ-dē-a
peptide PEP-tīd
phosphodiesterase fos′-fō-dī-ES-ter-ās
pineal PIN-ē-al
pinealocyte pin-ē-AL-ō-sīt
pituicyte pi-TOO-i-sīt
pituitary pi-TOO-i-tar′-ē

placenta   pla - SEN - ta
placental lactogen   pla - SEN - tal LAK - tō - gen
plexus   PLEK - sus
polypeptide   pol′ - ē - PEP - tīd
polyuria   pol′ - ē - YOO - rē - a
progesterone   prō - JES - te - rōn
prolactin   prō - LAK - tin
pro-opiomelanocortin   prō - ō′ - pē - ō - mel′ - an - ō - KOR - tin
prostaglandin   pros′ - ta - GLAN - din
protein   PRŌ - tēn
pubic symphysis   PYOO - bik   SIM - fi - sis
relaxin   rē - LAK - sin
renin   RĒ - nin
saccular   SAK - yoo - lar
secretin   sē - KRĒ - tin
sella turcica   SEL - a TUR - si - ca
somatomammotropin   sō′ - ma - tō - mam′ - ō - TRŌ - pin
somatomedin   sō′ - ma - tō - MĒ - din
somatostatin   sō′ - ma - tō - STAT - in
somatotroph   sō - MAT - ō - trōf
somatotropin   sō′ - ma - tō - TRŌ - pin
steroid   STER - oyd
supraopticohypophyseal   soo′ - pra - op′ - tik - ō - hī′ - pō - FIZ - ē - al
suprarenal   soo′ - pra - RĒ - nal
sympathomimetic   sim′ - pa - thō - mi - MET - ik
synergistic   sin - er - JIS - tik
testosterone   tes - TOS - te - rōn
thromboxane   throm - BOKS - ān
thymic   THĪ - mik
thymopoietin   thī′ - mō - POY - e - tin
thymosin   THĪ - mō - sin
thymus   THĪ - mus
thyroglobulin   thī - rō - GLOB - yoo - lin
thyroid   THĪ - royd
thyrotroph   THĪ - rō - trōf
thyrotropin   thī - rō - TRŌ - pin
thyroxine   thī - ROK - sin
triiodothyronine   trī - ī - ōd - ō - THĪ - rō - nēn
tropic   TRŌ - pik
tropin   TRŌ - pin
tyrosine   TĪ - rō - sēn
urea   yoo - RĒ - a
vasopressin   vas′ - ō - PRES - in
zona fasciculata   ZŌ - na fa - sik′ - yoo - LA - ta
zona glomerulosa   ZŌ - na glo - mer′ - yoo - LŌ - sa
zona reticularis   ZŌ - na ret - ik′ - yoo - LAR - is
zymogenic   zī′ - mō - JEN - ik

Glossary of Terms

Acetyl coenzyme A (acetyl CoA) A molecular complex that consists of an acetyl group (a 2-carbon fragment) and coenzyme A. In diabetes mellitus the production of ATP from fatty acids produces large quantities of acetyl coenzyme A as a by-product; the liver converts the excess acetyl coenzyme A into ketones, and this leads to acidosis.

Acidosis A condition in which blood pH is below 7.35. Also known as *acidemia*.

Acinar glands Exocrine glands whose pockets are shaped like sacs. Examples include the glands in the pancreas that secrete digestive enzymes, sebaceous glands, and salivary glands. Also called *saccular glands*.

Acromegaly A condition caused by hypersecretion (excessive secretion) of human growth hormone (hGH) during adulthood; it is characterized by thickened bones and the enlargement of other tissues.

Addison's disease A disorder caused by hyposecretion (diminished secretion) of the hormones cortisol and aldosterone; it is characterized by muscular weakness, hypoglycemia, mental lethargy, anorexia, nausea and vomiting, weight loss, low blood pressure, dehydration, and excessive skin and mucous membrane pigmentation.

Adenohypophysis *See* Anterior pituitary gland.

Adenylate cyclase An enzyme that converts ATP into cyclic AMP. It is located in plasma membranes and is activated when a hormone (or neurotransmitter) binds to its receptor.

Adrenal cortex The outer portion of an adrenal gland. It is divided into three zones : the zona fasciculata secretes cortisol; the zona glomerulosa secretes aldosterone; and the zona reticularis secretes sex hormones.

Adrenal glands Two glands, one above each kidney. Also called the *suprarenal glands*.

Adrenaline *See* Epinephrine.

Adrenal medulla The inner portion of an adrenal gland. It consists of modified postganglionic sympathetic neurons called chromaffin cells that secrete epinephrine and norepinephrine (NE) in response to the stimulation of preganglionic sympathetic neurons.

Adrenocorticotropic hormone (ACTH) A hormone secreted by the anterior pituitary gland; it acts on the adrenal cortex, stimulating the secretion of cortisol and aldosterone. Also called *adrenocorticotropin* and *corticotropin*.

Adrenocorticotropin *See* Adrenocorticotropic hormone.

Affinity Strength with which a ligand binds to its binding site, based on how well the complimentary shapes fit together and on how strong the forces of electrical attraction are.

Alarm reaction Activation of the sympathetic nervous system in response to stress. It is an immediate response to stress; a slower but longer lasting response involves the actions of certain hormones, and is called the resistance reaction. Also called the *fight-or-flight response*.

Aldosterone A hormone secreted by the adrenal cortex; it acts on the kidneys, promoting the retention of sodium (and therefore of water) and the excretion of potassium.

Allosteric modulation A modulator molecule binds to one binding site (the regulatory site) of a receptor; this alters the shape of a second binding site (the functional site).

Alpha cells Endocrine cells in the pancreatic islets that secrete the hormone glucagon when stimulated by low blood glucose levels.

Androgen Any hormone with testosterone-like actions.

Angiotensin I A protein produced by the action of the enzyme renin on angiotensinogen.

Angiotensin II A hormone that stimulates the adrenal cortex to secrete aldosterone. Angiotensin II is also a powerful vasoconstrictor. Both actions of angiotensin II tend to elevate the blood pressure.

Angiotensin converting enzyme (ACE) A plasma enzyme present in the lungs that converts angiotensin I into angiotensin II.

Angiotensinogen A plasma protein produced by the liver. The enzyme renin converts angiotensinogen into angiotensin I.

Antagonistic hormones Two hormones that have opposite effects on the same target cells. For example, insulin stimulates the uptake of glucose by liver cells (lowers blood glucose levels); glucagon stimulates the release of glucose by liver cells (elevates blood glucose levels).

Anterior hypophyseal veins Vessels that carry blood (and hormones) away from the anterior pituitary gland toward target cells.

Anterior pituitary gland Anterior portion (lobe) of the pituitary gland. Also called the *adenohypophysis*.

Antidiuretic hormone (ADH) A hormone secreted by the posterior pituitary gland. It promotes the retention of water by the kidneys, vasoconstriction of arteries, and a decrease in the cardiac output. Also called *vasopressin*.

Apocrine secretion A mechanism by which hormones are secreted by endocrine cells. It involves the breaking away of the entire top portion of a gland cell, releasing large numbers of Golgi vesicles into the extracellular fluid.

Arachidonic acid A 20-carbon fatty acid from which eicosanoids (prostaglandins and leukotrienes) are derived.

Atrial natriuretic peptide (ANP) A hormone secreted by cardiac muscle fibers of the atria in response to stretching. It increases sodium and water excretion in the urine (natriuresis and diuresis) and dilates blood vessels; both actions tend to decrease the blood pressure.

Autocrine A local hormone that acts on the same cell from which it has been secreted. An example is the hormone interleukin-2; after being released by a certain type of white blood cell (T cell), it binds to receptors on the plasma membrane of the same cell, stimulating mitosis.

Basal metabolic rate The rate of oxygen consumption at rest after an overnight fast. It is regulated mainly by thyroid hormones and epinephrine.

Basal rate of secretion The normal rate of secretion of any gland. The rate of secretion can be increased or decreased by stimulation from hormones or nerves.

Beta cells Endocrine cells in the pancreatic islets that secrete the hormone insulin when stimulated by high blood glucose levels.

Binding site The region of a protein to which a specific ligand binds.

Biogenic amines   A chemical classification for hormones. Hormones in this group include thyroid hormones, catecholamines (epinephrine and norepinephrine), and histamine.

Bound fraction   The 90 to 99.9% of water-insoluble hormones that are bound to plasma proteins while being transported in the blood.

Bound hormones   Hormones that are insoluble in water and must be bound to plasma proteins to make them water-soluble. They include thyroid hormones and steroids.

Calcitonin (CT)   A hormone secreted by the parafollicular cells of the thyroid gland. It lowers the calcium and phosphate levels of the blood by inhibiting bone breakdown and accelerating calcium absorption by bones.

Calcitriol   A hormone synthesized and secreted by the kidneys and produced in the skin by ultraviolet light. It stimulates the absorption of dietary calcium and phosphorus in the intestine; it increases the reabsorption of calcium by the kidneys. Its actions increase the levels of calcium and phosphorus in the blood. Also called *1, 25-dihydroxy cholecalciferol* and *1, 25-dihydroxy vitamin D_3*.

Calorigenic effect   The increase in the body temperature that results from an increase in the metabolic rate. Metabolic rate is controlled mainly by thyroid hormones and epinephrine.

Catabolism   Chemical reactions in cells that break down complex organic compounds into simpler ones with the release of energy.

Catecholamines   A class of chemicals that includes epinephrine, norepinephrine, and dopamine. All have similar chemical structures.

C (clear) cells   *See* Parafollicular cells.

Chemical messengers   Chemicals used for communication between cells and for communication inside a cell. Hormones, neurotransmitters, and second messengers (such as cyclic AMP) are all chemical messengers.

Chief cell   A secretory cell of a gastric gland in the stomach. It secretes pepsinogen (precursor of the enzyme pepsin) and the enzyme gastric lipase. (Principal cells of the parathyroid glands that secrete parathyroid hormone are also called chief cells.) Also called a *zymogenic cell.*

Cholecystokinin (CCK)   A hormone secreted by enteroendocrine cells located in the lining of the small intestine. It causes the gallbladder to contract, releasing bile into the duodenum; it stimulates the secretion of digestive enzymes by the pancreas; it stimulates the secretion of enterokinase, an enzyme released by cells lining the duodenum (enterokinase activates trypsinogen).

Cholesterol   A lipid that is the precursor for steroid hormones and bile salts. A component of plasma membranes.

Chromaffin cells   Sympathetic postganglionic neurons located in the adrenal medulla that are specialized to secrete epinephrine and norepinephrine.

Circulating hormones   Hormones that diffuse into the blood and act on distant target cells. Also called *endocrines.*

Colloid   The glutinous liquid that fills the lumen of a thyroid follicle, where thyroid hormones are synthesized.

Colony-stimulating factor (CSF)   One of a group of hematopoietins that stimulates development of white blood cells. Examples are macrophage CSF and granulocyte CSF.

Corticosterone   One of the three major glucocorticoids secreted by the zona fasciculata of the adrenal cortex. Along with the other two glucocorticoids (cortisol and cortisone) it regulates metabolism, provides resistance to stress, and inhibits the cells and secretions that participate in the inflammatory responses.

Corticotrophs   Endocrine cells in the anterior pituitary gland that secrete adrenocorticotropic hormone (ACTH) and melanocyte-stimulating hormone (MSH).

Corticotropin   *See* Adrenocorticotropic hormone.

Corticotropin-releasing hormone (CRH)   A hormone secreted by neurons in the hypothalamus. It stimulates cells (corticotrophs) in the anterior pituitary to secrete adrenocorticotropic hormone.

Cortisol   One of the three major glucocorticoids secreted by the zona fasciculata of the adrenal cortex. Along with the other two glucocorticoids (cortisone and corticosterone) it regulates metabolism, provides resistance to stress, and inhibits the cells and secretions that participate in the inflammatory responses. Cortisol is the most abundant of the glucocorticoids and is responsible for about 95% of glucocorticoid activity. Also called *hydrocortisone.*

Cortisone   One of the three major glucocorticoids secreted by the zona fasciculata of the adrenal cortex. Along with the other two glucocorticoids (cortisol and corticosterone) it regulates metabolism, provides resistance to stress, and inhibits the cells and secretions that participate in the inflammatory responses.

Cretinism   A condition caused by hyposecretion (undersecretion) of thyroid hormones during childhood. It is congenital and leads to mental and physical retardation.

Cushing's syndrome   A condition caused by hypersecretion (oversecretion) of cortisol and aldosterone. It is characterized by spindly legs, "moon face," "buffalo hump," pendulous abdomen, flushed facial skin, poor wound healing, hyperglycemia, osteoporosis, weakness, hypertension, and increased susceptibility to disease.

Cyclic AMP (cAMP)   A molecule formed from ATP by the action of the enzyme adenylate cyclase; it serves as an intracellular messenger (second messenger) for some hormones.

Cytokines   Growth factors that are secreted by lymphocytes, monocytes, macrophages, fibroblasts, and endothelial cells. They act primarily as local hormones (autocrines and paracrines) and have various roles in immunity and blood cell development.

Cytosol   The semifluid portion of the cytoplasm in which organelles and inclusions are suspended and solutes are dissolved. Also called *intracellular fluid.*

Degrading enzymes   Enzymes that break down (catabolize) hormones, resulting in their inactivation.

Delta cells (D-cells)   Endocrine cells in the pancreatic islets that secrete the hormone insulin when stimulated by high blood glucose levels.

Diabetes insipidus   A condition caused by hyposecretion (undersecretion) of antidiuretic hormone (ADH). It is characterized by thirst and the excretion of large amounts of urine (polyurea).

Diabetes mellitus   A condition caused by hyposecretion (undersecretion) of insulin. It is characterized by excessive thirst, high blood glucose levels (hyperglycemia), increased dilute urine production, glucose in the urine (glycosuria), excessive eating, and acidosis. It is hereditary.

Diencephalon A part of the brain consisting primarily of the thalamus and hypothalamus.

Diffusion A passive process in which there is a net or greater movement of molecules or ions from a region of high concentration to a region of low concentration until equilibrium is reached.

Dihydrotestosterone The active form of testosterone in certain of its target cells; formed by the alteration of testosterone by enzymes located on the target cells.

Dihydroxy cholecalciferol *See* Calcitriol.

Dihydroxy vitamin D$_3$ *See* Calcitriol.

Down-regulation Phenomenon in which there is a decrease in the number of receptors in response to an excess of a hormone or neurotransmitter.

Dwarfism *See* Pituitary dwarfism.

Eicosanoids A class of hormones. Two major types of eicosanoids are prostaglandins and leukotrienes. They are important local hormones, but they may also act as circulating hormones.

Electrolyte Any compound that separates into ions when dissolved in water and is able to conduct electricity.

Endocrine gland A gland that secretes hormones into the blood; a ductless gland.

Endocrines *See* Circulating hormones.

Endocrine system Endocrine glands and endocrine tissue contained in organs that are not endocrine glands exclusively.

Endocrine tissue Includes hormone-secreting cells found in endocrine glands and hormone-secreting cells found in structures other than endocrine glands. Many structures, such as the stomach and the pancreas, contain hormone-secreting cells, but they have other nonendocrine functions as well.

Endocrinology The science concerned with the structures and functions of endocrine glands and the diagnosis and treatment of the endocrine system.

Enteroendocrine cell Hormone-secreting cells that are scattered among the epithelial cells that line the inner walls of the digestive tract.

Epidermal growth factor (EGF) A growth factor that is produced in the submaxillary glands (salivary glands). It stimulates the proliferation of epithelial cells, fibroblasts, neurons, and astrocytes. It suppresses some cancer cells and the secretion of gastric juice by the stomach.

Epinephrine A hormone secreted by chromaffin cells in the adrenal medulla. Its actions mimic the responses that result from sympathetic stimulation (the physiological responses collectively called the fight-or-flight response). Also called *adrenaline*.

Epiphysis cerebri Pineal gland.

Erythropoiesis The process by which erythrocytes (red blood cells) are formed in the red bone marrow.

Erythropoietin A hormone released by the kidneys and liver in response to low blood oxygen concentrations. It stimulates an increased production of erythrocytes (red blood cells) in red bone marrow.

Estrogens Female sex hormones secreted by maturing granulosa (follicle) cells in the ovaries. These hormones are concerned with the development and maintenance of female reproductive structures, secondary sex characteristics, fluid and electrolyte balance, and protein anabolism. Examples are beta-estradiol, estrone, and estriol.

Exhaustion A condition caused by loss of potassium (cells dehydrate), depletion of cortisol (blood glucose levels drop), and weakened organs.

Exocrine gland Glands that secrete to the outside of the body. Their secretions flow through ducts to the epithelial surface, which is either the skin or the lining of a hollow organ.

Exocytosis A process of discharging cellular products too big to go through the membrane. Particles for export are enclosed by Golgi membranes when they are synthesized. Vesicles pinch off from the Golgi complex and carry the enclosed particles to the interior surface of the cell membrane, where the vesicle membrane and plasma membrane fuse and the contents of the vesicle are discharged.

F-cells Endocrine cells in the pancreatic islets that secrete the hormone pancreatic polypeptide.

Fibroblast growth factor (FGF) A growth factor found in the pituitary gland and the brain. It stimulates the proliferation of many cells derived from embryonic mesoderm (fibroblasts, adrenocortical cells, smooth muscle fibers, chondrocytes, and endothelial cells); it also stimulates cell migration and growth and production of the adhesion protein and fibronectin.

Fight-or-flight response *See* Alarm reaction.

First messenger When more than one chemical messenger is involved in altering a cell's activities, the hormone or neurotransmitter is referred to as the first messenger. Chemical messengers inside the cell, such as cyclic AMP, are referred to as second messengers.

Follicle A small, fluid-filled, secretory sac or cavity.

Follicle-stimulating hormone (FSH) A hormone secreted by cells (gonadotrophs) in the anterior pituitary. In females it initiates the development of ova (eggs) and stimulates the ovaries to secrete estrogens; in males it initiates sperm production.

Free fraction The 0.1 to 10% of water-insoluble hormones that do not bind to plasma proteins while being transported by the blood.

"Free" hormones Water-soluble hormones that circulate "free" in the plasma (unbound to plasma proteins). Free, water-soluble hormones include epinephrine, norepinephrine, and peptide hormones.

Functional site A binding site on an allosteric receptor protein. When a modulator molecule binds to the regulatory site of the receptor, it causes a change in the shape of the functional site, making it receptive to a ligand.

Gastric inhibitory peptide (GIP) A hormone secreted by enteroendocrine cells of the intestinal lining in response to the presence of glucose and fat in the duodenum. It inhibits motility of the stomach and the secretion of gastric juices.

Gastrin A hormone secreted by G-cells in the lining of the stomach in response to the presence of partially digested proteins in the stomach and to distension of the stomach. It stimulates the secretion of gastric juice, causes contraction of the lower esophageal sphincter, increases the motility of the stomach, and relaxes the pyloric sphincter and ileocecal sphincter.

G-cells Endocrine cells located in the lining of the pyloric antrum of the stomach that secrete the hormone gastrin.

Gene A unit of hereditary information located in a definite position on a particular chromosome. A portion of a DNA molecule that contains the information required to determine the amino acid sequence for a particular protein.

General adaptation syndrome (GAS)   A wide-ranging set of bodily changes triggered by a stressor. It gears the body to meet an emergency.

Giantism   *See* Pituitary giantism.

Gland   A single epithelial cell or group of epithelial cells that secrete substances into ducts, onto a surface, or into the blood.

Glucagon   A hormone secreted by the alpha cells of the pancreatic islets in response to decreased concentrations of glucose in the blood. It causes an increase in blood glucose levels.

Glucocorticoids   Hormones secreted by the adrenal cortex that influence glucose metabolism (especially the hormone cortisol).

Gluconeogenesis   The conversion of a substance other than carbohydrate into glucose.

Glycogenesis   The process by which many molecules of glucose combine to form a molecule called glycogen, a storage form of glucose found mostly in liver and skeletal muscle cells.

Glycogenolysis   The process of converting glycogen into glucose. Glycogen catabolism.

Glycosuria   The presence of glucose in the urine; may be temporary or pathological. Also called *glucosuria*.

Gonad   An organ that produces gametes (sperm or eggs) and hormones (sex hormones); the testes in the male and the ovaries in the female.

Gonadocorticoids   Sex hormones secreted by the zona reticularis of the adrenal cortex.

Gonadotrophs   Endocrine cells located in the anterior pituitary gland that secrete follicle-stimulating hormone (FSH) and luteinizing hormone (LH).

Gonadotropin-releasing hormone (GnRH)   A hormone secreted by neurons in the hypothalamus. It stimulates cells (gonadotrophs) in the anterior pituitary gland to release follicle-stimulating hormone (FSH) and luteinizing hormone (LH).

G-protein   A regulatory protein found in the plasma membrane that responds when a receptor on the outer surface of the membrane is activated. When activated, the G - protein alters the permeability of membrane ion channels or activates enzymes inside the cell, such as adenylate cyclase.

Grave's disease   A condition caused by hypersecretion (oversecretion) of thyroid hormones. It is characterized by an increased metabolic rate and heart rate.

Growth factors   Peptide hormones that are highly effective in stimulating the growth, mitosis, and differentiation of certain cell types. More than forty of these recently discovered hormones have been described; many act locally as autocrines and paracrines.

Growth hormone (GH)   *See* Human growth hormone.

Growth hormone-inhibiting hormone (GHIH) A hormone secreted by neurons in the hypothalamus; it inhibits the release of human growth hormone (hGH) by cells in the anterior pituitary gland. GHIH is also secreted by D-cells in pancreatic islets; it acts as a paracrine to inhibit the secretion of insulin and glucagon by the pancreas. Also called *somatostatin*.

Growth hormone-releasing hormone (GHRH) A hormone secreted by neurons in the hypothalamus. It stimulates cells in the anterior pituitary gland to release human growth hormone (hGH). Also called *somatocrinin*.

Half-life   The time after secretion of a peptide hormone for half of the hormones to be inactivated. For example, the half-life for insulin is about 5 minutes.

Hematopoietic growth factors   Local hormones involved in blood cell formation (hematopoiesis).

Histamine   A substance found in many cells, especially mast cells, basophils, and platelets. When the cells are injured it is released, causing vasodilation and increased permeability of local blood vessels; it also causes the constriction of bronchiole tubes. Histamine is an example of an paracrine, because it acts on nearby cells.

Histidine   The amino acid from which histamine is derived.

Holocrine secretion   A mechanism by which hormones are secreted by endocrine cells. It involves the complete disintegration of the gland cell; all of the contents are released at once and the cell is destroyed. The cells of sebaceous (oil) glands function in this way.

Homeostasis   The relative stability of the internal environment (extracellular fluid). It results from the action of feedback systems (reflex arcs), which constantly monitor changes and make adjustments by negative feedback.

Hormone   A secretion of an endocrine tissue that is released into the bloodstream, combines with the receptors of specific target cells, and alters a specific cell function.

Hormone receptor   A protein molecule that has a binding site for a specific hormone. Receptors for peptide hormones are located on the outer surface of plasma membranes; receptors for steroid hormones are located in the cytosol.

Human chorionic gonadotropin (hCG)   A hormone secreted by the chorion of the placenta. It maintains the activity of the corpus luteum during the first three months of pregnancy.

Human chorionic somatomammotropin (hCS) A hormone secreted by the chorion of the placenta. It stimulates breast tissue for lactation, enhances body growth, and regulates metabolism. Also called *human placental lactogen (hPL)*.

Human growth hormone (hGH)   A hormone secreted by cells (somatotrophs) in the anterior pituitary gland. It brings about growth of body tissues, especially skeletal and muscular. Also known as *growth hormone, somatotropin* and *somatotropic hormone (STH)*.

Hydrochloric acid (HCl)   An acid secreted into the lumen of the stomach by parietal cells. Secretion of HCl is stimulated by the hormone gastrin.

Hydrogen ion (H$^+$)   Proton. The concentration of hydrogen ions determines the acidity of a solution. Blood concentration of H$^+$ is maintained at a relatively constant level by the homeostatic actions of the hormone aldosterone.

Hypercalcemia   An elevated blood calcium level.

Hyperglycemia   An elevated blood sugar level.

Hypersecretion   Overactivity of glands resulting in excessive secretion.

Hypertension   High blood pressure.

Hypertonic   Having an osmotic pressure greater than that of a solution with which it is compared.

Hypocalcemia   Below normal level of calcium in the blood.

Hypoglycemia   Below normal level of glucose in the blood.

Hypokalemia   Below normal level of potassium in the blood.

Hyponatremia   Below normal level of sodium in the blood.

Hypophyseal portal veins   Vessels that carry blood from the primary plexus (in the base of the hypothalamus) down the infundibulum (stalk of the pituitary gland) to the secondary plexus in the anterior pituitary. These vessels carry releasing and inhibiting hormones from the hypothalamus to their target cells in the anterior pituitary gland.

Hypophysiotropic hormones Releasing and inhibiting hormones secreted by neurons in the hypothalamus that act on the hypophysis (pituitary gland).

Hypophysis The pituitary gland.

Hyposecretion Underactivity of glands resulting in diminished secretion.

Hypothalamus A portion of the diencephalon (in the brain). It lies beneath the two lobes of the thalamus, forming the floor and part of the walls of the third ventricle. It consists of about 12 nuclei that play an important role in regulating the internal environment. Neurons in the hypothalamus secrete tropic hormones that inhibit or stimulate the release of hormones by the anterior pituitary gland; two hormones, oxytocin and antidiuretic hormone, are produced by neurons in the hypothalamus and are secreted by their axon terminals, which are located in the posterior pituitary gland.

Hypotonic Having an osmotic pressure lower than that of a solution with which it is compared.

I-cell Endocrine cells in the lining of the upper portion of the small intestine that secrete the hormone cholecystokinin (CCK).

IGF-1 and IGF-2 *See* Insulinlike growth factor.

IL *See* Interleukin-1 and Interleukin-2.

Inferior hypophyseal arteries Blood vessels that supply the posterior pituitary gland. They form a capillary network called the plexus of the infundibular process.

Infundibulum The stalklike structure that attaches the pituitary gland to the hypothalamus of the brain. (Also the funnel-shaped, open, distal end of the uterine (Fallopian) tube.

Inhibin A hormone secreted by the gonads (ovaries and testes). It inhibits the release of FSH by cells (gonadotrophs) in the anterior pituitary gland.

Inhibiting hormones Hormones secreted by neurons in the hypothalamus that can suppress the secretion of hormones by the anterior pituitary gland.

Insulin A hormone secreted by the beta cells of the pancreatic islets in response to increased concentrations of glucose in the blood. It causes a decrease in the blood glucose level.

Insulinlike growth factor (IGF) One of a group of small protein hormones synthesized and released by the liver in response to stimulation by human growth hormone (hGH). Stimulates the growth of chondrocytes, fibroblasts, and other cells. Also called *somatomedin*.

Interferons (IFNs) Three types of small protein hormones (alpha, beta, and gamma) produced by virus-infected host cells. They induce nearby uninfected cells to synthesize antiviral proteins that inhibit viral replication.

Interleukin-1 (IL-1) A small protein hormone secreted by monocytes and macrophages that stimulates proliferation of B cells and T cells, increases the number of circulating neutrophils, stimulates production of immune substances by the liver, and induces fever.

Interleukin-2 (IL-2) A small protein hormone secreted by a type of lymphocyte (activated helper T cells). It stimulates the proliferation of other lymphocytes (cytotoxic T cells and B cells). It activates natural killer cells (NK cells). Also called the *T cell growth factor*.

Interstitial cell of Leydig *See* Interstitial endocrinocyte.

Interstitial cell-stimulating hormone (ICSH) A hormone secreted by cells (gonadotrophs) in the anterior pituitary gland of males. It stimulates the secretion of testosterone by the interstitial cells of Leydig (in the testes).

Interstitial endocrinocyte A cell located in the connective tissue between seminiferous tubules in a mature testis; it secretes the hormone testosterone. Also called an *interstitial cell of Leydig*.

Iodine trapping The active transport of iodide (I⁻) from the blood into the follicular cells of the thyroid gland. The iodide is needed for the synthesis of thyroid hormones.

Ion (electrolyte) Any charged particle or group of particles; usually formed when a substance, such as a salt, dissolves and dissociates in water. Positively charged ions are called cations; negatively charged ions are called anions.

Islets of Langerhans *See* Pancreatic islets.

Isotonic Having equal osmotic pressure between two different solutions.

Isthmus A narrow strip of tissue or a narrow passage connecting two larger parts.

Juxtaglomerular cells Specialized cells in the kidneys that secrete the enzyme renin in response to low blood pressure.

Ketone bodies Substances produced primarily during excessive triglyceride (fat) catabolism. Three substances (acetoacetic acid, hydroxybutyric acid, and acetone) are collectively known as ketone bodies. They lower the pH of body fluids and may cause acidosis. Also called *ketones*.

Ketosis Abnormal condition marked by excessive production of ketone bodies.

Kidney One of the paired organs located in the lumbar region that regulates the composition and volume of blood and produces urine.

Kidney stone A concretion (solid mass), usually consisting of calcium oxalate, uric acid, and calcium phosphate crystals, that may form in any portion of the urinary tract. Also called a *renal calculus*.

Lactation The secretion and ejection of milk by the mammary glands. Regulated by the hormones oxytocin and prolactin.

Lactogenic hormone *See* Prolactin.

Lactotrophs Endocrine cells in the anterior pituitary gland that secrete the hormone prolactin (PRL).

Lateral lobes The two lobes of the thyroid gland; located on each side of the trachea.

Leukotrienes (LTs) A family of eicosanoid molecules that act as local hormones (paracrines or autocrines) in most tissues of the body. They are synthesized from arachidonic acid (a fatty acid).

Ligand Any molecule or ion that attaches to a binding site of a protein receptor by noncovalent bonds.

Lipogenesis The synthesis of lipids from glucose or amino acids by liver cells. Stimulated by the hormone insulin.

Lipolysis The breakdown of triglycerides (fats) into fatty acids and glycerol. It occurs in adipose tissue and is stimulated by the hormone glucagon. Fat catabolism.

Liver A large gland under the diaphragm that occupies most of the right hypochondriac region and part of the epigastric region. Its many functions include : the production of bile salts, heparin, plasma proteins, and somatomedins; the conversion of one nutrient into another; the detoxification of substances; the storage of glycogen, minerals, and vitamins; the phagocytosis of blood cells and bacteria; and the activation of vitamin D.

Local hormones   Hormones that act locally. There are two types of local hormones : an autocrine acts on the same cell that secretes it; a paracrine acts on neaby cells.

Lumen   The space within an artery, vein, intestine, or tube.

Luteinizing hormone (LH)   A hormone secreted by cells (gonadotrophs) in the anterior pituitary gland. It stimulates ovulation and progesterone secretion by the corpus luteum; it readies the mammary glands for milk secretion in females; and stimulates testosterone secretion by the testes in males.

Lymphocyte   A type of white blood cell. There are two main classes of lymphocytes : B cells and T cells.

Lymphokines   Small protein hormones secreted by lymphocytes that act as local hormones (autocrines and paracrines). They are involved in various immune system responses.

Macrophage   A phagocytic cell derived from a monocyte.

Mammary gland   A modified sudoriferous (sweat) gland that secretes milk for the nourishment of the young.

Mast cell   A cell found in areolar connective tissue along blood vessels. During the inflammatory response it releases heparin and histamine, which cause the dilation of small blood vessels.

Median eminence   A region at the base of the hypothalamus. In this region tropic hormones are secreted from neuron axon terminals into a capillary network called the primary plexus.

Melanocyte   A pigmented cell located between or beneath cells of the deepest layer of the epidermis that synthesizes melanin.

Melanocyte-stimulating hormone (MSH)   A hormone secreted by cells in the anterior pituitary gland; its function is unknown.

Melatonin   A hormone produced during darkness by the pineal gland; its formation is interrupted when light enters the eyes and stimulates retinal neurons. Its function is unknown.

Metabolic rate   The total body energy expenditure per unit time. It is regulated by thyroid hormones.

Milk ejection reflex   The contraction of alveolar cells to force milk into ducts of mammary glands. It is stimulated by the hormone oxytocin (OT), which is released from the posterior pituitary gland in response to suckling action. Also called the *milk let-down reflex*.

Mineralocorticoids   A group of steroid hormones produced by the adrenal cortex; especially the hormone aldosterone. They regulate the sodium and potassium balance in the body fluids.

Mobilization   The process of making a stored substance mobile, causing its release into the circulation for body use, as in the mobilization of fats stored in adipose tissue.

Modulator molecule   A ligand that binds to a regulatory site on an allosteric receptor protein. When it binds to the regulatory site it alters the shape of another binding site on the receptor, the functional site, making it more or less receptive to a ligand.

Monocyte   A type of white blood cell (leukocyte); characterized by agranular cytoplasm.

Monokines   Small protein hormones secreted by monocytes or macrophages that act as local hormones (autocrines and paracrines). They are involved in various immune system responses.

MSH-inhibiting hormone (MIH)   A hormone secreted by neurons in the hypothalamus. It inhibits the release of melanocyte-stimulating hormone from the anterior pituitary gland.

MSH-releasing hormone (MRH)   A hormone secreted by neurons in the hypothalamus. It stimulates the release of melanocyte-stimulating hormone from the anterior pituitary gland.

Myxedema   A condition caused by the hyposecretion (undersecretion) of thyroid hormones during the adult years. It is characterized by the swelling of facial tissues, mental sluggishness, dry skin, and fatigue.

Negative feedback   The principle governing most control systems. It is a response mechanism in which the stimulus initiates actions that reverse or reduce the stimulus. This is the primary mechanism for maintaining homeostasis. The secretion of many types of hormones is regulated by negative feedback.

Nerve growth factor (NGF)   A growth factor produced in the submaxillary glands (salivary glands) and parts of the brain (hippocampus). It stimulates the growth of ganglia in embryonic life, maintains the sympathetic nervous system, and stimulates the hypertrophy (overgrowth) and differentiation of mature nerve cells.

Neuroendocrine reflex   A reflex that involves both nerves and hormones.

Neuroendocrine system   A term that suggests the close relationship that exists between the nervous and endocrine systems. The two systems are sometimes referred to as a single system because of their mutual functions of coordinating bodily activities and maintaining homeostasis. Certain parts of the nervous system control the secretion of hormones, and some hormones promote or inhibit the generation of nerve impulses.

Neurohormones   Hormones synthesized and secreted by neurons. Tropic hormones released by neurons in the hypothalamus are neurohormones.

Neurohypophysis   The posterior pituitary gland.

Neurosecretory cells   Neurons in the paraventricular and supraoptic nuclei of the hypothalamus that secrete the hormones oxytocin (OT) and antidiuretic hormone (ADH).

Neurotransmitters   Molecules that transmit impulses across synapses from a presynaptic neuron to a postsynaptic neuron or effector cell.

Noradrenaline   *See* Norepinephrine.

Norepinephrine   A hormone secreted by chromaffin cells in the adrenal medulla. Its actions mimic the responses that result from sympathetic stimulation (the physiological responses collectively called the fight-or-flight response). Also called *noradrenaline*.

Nucleoplasm   The fluid inside the nucleus of a cell.

Nutrient   A chemical substance in food that provides energy, forms new body components, or assists in the functioning of various body processes.

Osmoreceptors   Receptors in the hypothalamus that respond to high osmotic pressure (low water concentration). When activated they stimulate the neurosecretory cells of the supraoptic and paraventricular nuclei to synthesize and secrete antidiuretic hormone (ADH).

Osmotic diuresis   An increased excretion of water in the urine, resulting from an increased osmotic pressure in the urine. In diabetes mellitus an increased osmotic pressure in the urine is due to high concentrations of glucose.

Osteoclast A cell that destroys (or resorbs) bone tissue, increasing the release of calcium into the blood. Parathyroid hormone (PTH) stimulates osteoclasts.

Ovary The female gonad (reproductive organ). The two ovaries produce ova (eggs) and hormones (estrogens, progesterone, and relaxin).

Oxyphil cells One of the two types of cells found in the parathyroid glands; their function is unknown. Principal cells that secrete parathyroid hormone are the other type.

Oxytocin (OT) A hormone synthesized by neurons located in the paraventricular and supraoptic nuclei of the hypothalamus; the axon terminals from which it is secreted are located in the posterior pituitary gland. It stimulates the contraction of the smooth muscle fibers (cells) in the pregnant uterus and contractile cells around the ducts of mammary glands.

Pancreas A soft organ lying along the greater curvature of the stomach and connected by a duct to the duodenum. It is both exocrine (secreting pancreatic juice) and endocrine (secreting insulin, glucagon, growth hormone-inhibiting hormone, and pancreatic polypeptide).

Pancreatic islets Clusters of endocrine cells in the pancreas that secrete insulin, glucagon, growth hormone-inhibiting hormone, and pancreatic polypeptide. Also called *islets of Langerhans*.

Pancreatic polypeptide A hormone secreted by F-cells in the pancreatic islets. It regulates the release of pancreatic digestive enzymes.

Paracrines Hormones that act on nearby cells.

Parafollicular cells Cells that lie between the follicles in the thyroid gland; they secrete the hormone calcitonin (CT), which decreases blood calcium levels. Also called *C cells* or *clear cells*.

Parathormone *See* Parathyroid hormone.

Parathyroid gland One of four small endocrine glands embedded on the posterior surfaces of the lateral lobes of the thyroid gland. Principal cells (chief cells) of the parathyroid glands secrete parathyroid hormone (PTH).

Parathyroid hormone (PTH) A hormone secreted by the principal (chief) cells of the parathyroid glands in response to decreased concentrations of calcium in the blood. It increases the blood calcium level and decreases the blood phosphate level. Also called *parathormone*.

Pars intermedia A small avascular zone between the anterior and posterior pituitary glands.

Pepsinogen The inactive form of pepsin. When stimulated by the hormone gastrin, chief cells of the stomach secrete pepsinogen. Pepsinogen is converted into pepsin (a protein-digesting enzyme) by hydrochloric acid.

Peptide Any molecule consisting of two or more amino acids. Peptides form the constituent parts of proteins.

Permissive effect A hormonal interaction in which the effect of one hormone on a target cell requires previous or simultaneous exposure to another hormone(s). For example, previous exposure of the uterus to estrogen enhances the effect of progesterone in preparing the lining of the uterus for implantation.

pH A symbol for the concentration of hydrogen ions in a solution. The pH scale extends from 0 to 14. A pH of 7 indicates neutrality; values lower than 7 indicate increasing acidity; values higher than 7 indicate increasing alkalinity.

phagocytosis The process by which cells (phagocytes) ingest particulate matter; especially the ingestion and destruction of microbes, cell debris, and other foreign matter.

Phosphodiesterase An enzyme present in the cytosol of cells that inactivates cyclic AMP (second messenger), turning off a cell's response to a hormone.

Pineal gland The cone-shaped gland located in the roof of the third ventricle of the brain. It secretes the hormone melatonin, whose function is unknown. Also called the *epiphysis cerebri*.

Pinealocyte An endocrine cell in the pineal gland that secretes the hormone melatonin.

Pituicytes A supporting cell in the posterior pituitary gland. It supports the axon terminals of the neurons that secrete oxytocin and antidiuretic hormone.

Pituitary dwarfism A condition caused by hyposecretion (undersecretion) of human growth hormone (hGH) during the growth years. It is characterized by childlike physical traits in an adult. Also called *dwarfism*.

Pituitary giantism A condition caused by the hypersecretion (oversecretion) of human growth hormone (hGH) during childhood. It is characterized by a large body size and normal proportions. Also called *giantism* and *gigantism*.

Pituitary gland A small endocrine gland lying in the sella turcica (Turk's saddle) of the sphenoid bone. It is attached to the hypothalamus by a stalk called the infundibulum. It consists of two lobes : the anterior pituitary gland and the posterior pituitary gland. Also called the *hypophysis*.

Placenta The special structure through which the exchange of materials between fetal and maternal circulations occurs. It secretes several hormones : human chorionic gonadotropin, human chorionic somatomammotropin, relaxin, estrogen, and progesterone. Also called the *afterbirth*.

Platelet-derived growth factor (PDGF) A growth factor produced in blood platelets. It stimulates the proliferation of several cell types, including neuroglia, smooth muscle fibers, and fibroblasts. It appears to have a role in wound healing, and it may contribute to the development of atherosclerosis.

Plexus A network of blood vessels, lymphatic vessels, or nerves.

Plexus of the infundibular process A network of capillaries located in the posterior pituitary gland and formed by the inferior hypophyseal arteries. The hormones oxytocin and antidiuretic hormone are released into these capillaries.

Polyuria An excessive production of urine.

Posterior hypophyseal veins Blood vessels that carry hormones out of the posterior pituitary gland for distribution to tissue cells.

Posterior pituitary gland The posterior portion (lobe) of the pituitary gland. Also called the *neurohypophysis*.

Primary plexus A capillary network at the base of the hypothalamus. Releasing and inhibiting hormones secreted by hypothalamic neurons diffuse into the capillaries of this plexus.

Principal cells Endocrine cells in the parathyroid glands that secrete parathyroid hormone. (Also the cells found in the distal convoluted tubules and collecting ducts of kidney nephrons). The principal cells of parathyroid glands are also called *chief cells*.

Progesterone (PROG) A hormone secreted by granulosa

cells in ovarian follicles and by luteal cells of the corpus luteum. It prepares the uterine lining and mammary glands for pregnancy.

Prohormones Large peptides that are the precursors of peptide hormones. They are split by enzymes to form fragments that are the active hormones.

Prolactin (PRL) A hormone secreted by cells (lactotrophs) in the anterior pituitary gland. It initiates and maintains milk secretion by the mammary glands. Also called *lactogenic hormone*.

Prolactin-inhibiting hormone (PIH) A hormone secreted by neurons in the hypothalamus. It inhibits the release of prolactin from cells (lactotrophs) in the anterior pituitary gland.

Prolactin-releasing hormone (PRH) A hormone secreted by neurons in the hypothalamus. It stimulates the release of prolactin from cells (lactotrophs) in the anterior pituitary gland.

Pro-opiomelanocortin (POMC) A large protein precursor molecule synthesized by corticotrophs in the anterior pituitary gland. ACTH and MSH are split from POMC.

Prostaglandins (PGs) A family of eicosanoid molecules that act as local hormones (paracrines or autocrines) in most tissues of the body. They are synthesized from arachidonic acid (a fatty acid).

Prostate gland A doughnut-shaped gland inferior to the urinary bladder that surrounds the superior portion of the male urethra. It secretes a slightly acid solution that contributes to sperm motility and viability.

Protein An organic compound consisting of carbon, hydrogen, oxygen, nitrogen, and sometimes sulfur and phosphorus. Proteins are made up of amino acids linked by peptide bonds. The great majority of all hormones are proteins or peptides.

Protein kinases One of a family of enzymes that phosphorylates (adds a phosphate group) to a particular protein. The phosphate group is transferred from a molecule of ATP.

Pubic symphysis A slightly movable cartilaginous joint between the anterior surfaces of the hipbones.

Receptor Biological receptors are of two types. In chemical communication, a receptor is a protein in the plasma membrane or in the cytosol of the target cell; a chemical messenger combines with a specific binding site on the receptor protein. In the sensory system, a receptor is a cell that is sensitive to a particular type of stimulus.

Receptor modulation A change in the shape of the binding site in a protein receptor. When a modulator molecule or a phosphate group attaches to a receptor protein, it alters the distribution of forces within the protein, and this may alter (modulate) the shape of a binding site on that protein.

Regulatory site The binding site on an allosteric receptor protein to which a modulator molecule attaches. When a modulator molecule attaches to a regulatory site, another binding site called the functional site changes shape, and becomes more receptive to its ligand.

Relaxin (RLX) A hormone secreted by the ovaries and placenta. It relaxes the pubic symphysis and helps dilate the uterine cervix to ease delivery of a baby.

Releasing hormones Neurohormones secreted by neurons in the hypothalamus. They stimulate the release of hormones from cells in the anterior pituitary gland.

Renin An enzyme released by the kidneys into the blood plasma. In the blood it converts angiotensinogen into angiotensin 1.

Renin-angiotensin pathway A mechanism for the control of aldosterone secretion. It is initiated by secretion of renin by the kidneys in response to low blood pressure.

Resistance reaction A response to stress that is initiated by regulating hormones (CRH, GHRH, and TRH) secreted by the hypothalamus. The response is slow, but long-lasting. Catabolism is accelerated to provide energy to counteract the stress; ACTH stimulates the adrenal cortex to secrete cortisol, which raises the blood glucose level, and aldosterone, which raises the blood pressure.

Sebaceous gland An exocrine gland usually associated with a hair follicle of the skin; secretes sebum. Also called an *oil gland*.

Secondary plexus A capillary network in the inferior portion of the infundibulum (stalk of the pituitary gland). It receives blood from the hypophyseal portal veins that are carrying releasing and inhibiting hormones from the hypothalamus; these hormones stimulate the release of anterior pituitary hormones, which diffuse into the secondary plexus and are carried out of the anterior pituitary gland via the anterior hypophyseal veins.

Second messenger An intracellular substance that increases as a result of the binding of the first messenger to its receptor in the plasma membrane. The second messenger serves as a relay from the plasma membrane to the inside of the cell, where it alters a particular cell activity. The best known second messenger is cyclic AMP.

Secretin A hormone secreted by enteroendocrine cells located in the upper portion of the small intestine in response to partially digested proteins and a low (acidic) pH. It stimulates the secretion of bicarbonate ions by the pancreas and liver.

Secretion The production and release of organic molecules, ions, and water by gland cells in response to a specific stimulus.

Sella turcica A depression on the superior surface of the sphenoid bone that houses the pituitary gland. In Latin, sella turcica means *Turk's saddle*.

Sex hormones The male sex hormone is testosterone. The female sex hormones are estrogens and progesterone.

Small intestine A long tube of the gastrointestinal tract about 1 inch in diameter and 21 feet in length. It begins at the pyloric sphincter of the stomach, coils through the central and lower part of the abdominal cavity, and ends at the large intestine. It is divided into three segments : duodenum, jejunum, and ileum.

Somatocrinin *See* Growth hormone-releasing hormone.

Somatomedin A small protein produced by the liver in response to stimulation by human growth hormone (hGH). It mediates most of the effects of hGH. Also called *insulin-like growth factor*.

Somatostatin *See* Growth hormone-inhibiting hormone.

Somatotrophs Endocrine cells in the anterior pituitary gland that secrete human growth hormone (hGH).

Somatotropin *See* Human growth hormone.

Steroid A subclass of lipids. All lipids consist of four interconnected carbon rings to which polar groups may be attached.

Stomach The J-shaped enlargement of the gastrointestinal tract directly under the diaphragm in the epigastric, umbilical, and left hypochondriac regions of the abdomen, between the esophagus and small intestine.

Stressor A stress that is extreme, unusual, or long-lasting and triggers the stress response (general adaptation syndrome).

Stress response A wide-ranging set of bodily changes that prepare the body to meet an emergency. The stress response involves two pathways : the alarm reaction (or fight-or-flight response) is a complex of reactions initiated by hypothalamic stimulation of the sympathetic nervous system and the adrenal medulla. The resistance reaction is initiated by hypothalamic hormones; it is a slower, longer-lasting response. Also called the *general adaptation syndrome (GAS)*.

Substrate A substance with which an enzyme reacts.

Sudoriferous gland A gland in the dermis or subcutaneous layer of the skin that produces perspiration. Also called a *sweat gland*.

Superior hypophyseal arteries Branches of the internal carotid and posterior communicating arteries; they carry blood into the capillary network known as the primary plexus, which is located at the base of the hypothalamus.

Supraopticohypophyseal tract Nerve fibers that extend from the hypothalamus to the posterior pituitary; they have their cell bodies in the hypothalamus but release their secretions (oxytocin and antidiuretic hormone) in the posterior pituitary gland.

Sympathomimetic Producing effects that mimic those brought about by the sympathetic division of the autonomic nervous system.

Synergistic effect A hormonal interaction in which the effects of two or more hormones complement each other; the target cell responds to the sum of the hormones involved. An example is the combined actions of estrogens, progesterone, prolactin, and oxytocin; all of the these hormones act on the breasts to regulate lactation.

Target cell A cell whose activity is affected by a particular hormone.

T cell A subclass of lymphocytes. Lymphocytes are one of the five major types of white blood cells. Also called *T lymphocytes*.

Testis (plural : testes) The male gonad (reproductive gland). It produces sperm and the hormones testosterone and inhibin. Also called a *testicle*.

Testosterone The principal androgen (male sex hormone). It is secreted by the interstitial cells of Leydig in the testes. It controls the growth, development, and maintenance of sex organs; stimulates bone growth, protein anabolism, and sperm maturation; and stimulates development of the male secondary sex characteristics.

Thromboxane (TX) A modified prostaglandin that constricts blood vessels and stimulates platelet aggregation and secretion of platelet granules during blood clotting.

Thymic hormones Hormones involved in immune responses that are secreted by the thymus gland. Thymosin, thymic humoral factor (THF), thymic factor (TF), and thymopoietin promote the maturation of T cells (a type of lymphocyte).

Thymus gland An organ consisting of two lobes (bilobed) located posterior to the sternum and between the lungs in the anterior part of the superior mediastinum. It plays an essential role in the immune mechanism of the body. Hormones produced by the thymus promote the proliferation and maturation of T cells, which destroy foreign microbes and substances.

Thyroglobulin (TGB) A large, glycoprotein molecule produced by follicle cells of the thyroid gland, and then released by exocytosis into the lumen of the follicle. Thyroid hormones are synthesized within thyroglobulin from iodine and the amino acid tyrosine.

Thyroid follicles Spherical sacs that form the functional tissues of the thyroid gland. They consist of follicular cells that produce triiodothyronine (T_3) and thyroxine (T_4) and parafollicular cells that produce calcitonin (CT).

Thyroid gland An endocrine gland with right and left lateral lobes on either side of the trachea just below the thyroid cartilage (Adam's apple).

Thyroid hormones (TH) The two hormones secreted by the follicles in the thyroid gland : triiodothyronine (T_3) and thyroxine (T_4). They increase the metabolic rate and the cardiac output.

Thyroid-stimulating hormone (TSH) A hormone secreted by cells (thyrotrophs) in the anterior pituitary gland. It stimulates the thyroid gland to release the thyroid hormones, triiodothyronine (T_3) and thyroxine (T_4). Also called *thyrotropin*.

Thyrotrophs Endocrine cells in the anterior pituitary gland that secrete thyroid-stimulating hormone (TSH).

Thyrotropin *See* Thyroid–stimulating hormone.

Thyrotropin-releasing hormone (TRH) A hormone secreted by neurons in the hypothalamus. It stimulates cells (thyrotrophs) in the anterior pituitary gland to release thyroid–stimulating hormone (TSH).

Thyroxine (T_4) *See* Thyroid hormones.

Thyroxine-binding globulin (TBG) A transport protein that combines with the thyroid hormones, making them water-soluble for transport in the blood.

Transport proteins Plasma proteins synthesized by the liver that combine with lipid-soluble (water-insoluble) steroid and thyroid hormones. They improve the transportability of the lipid-soluble hormones by making them temporarily water-soluble; they retard the loss of the small hormone molecules through the filtering mechanism in the kidneys, thus slowing the hormone loss in the urine; and they provide a ready reserve of hormone already present in the blood.

Triiodothyronine (T_3) *See* Thyroid hormones.

Tropic hormones Hormones that regulate the secretion of other hormones. For example, thyroid-stimulating hormone (TSH) is secreted by cells in the anterior pituitary and it stimulates the release of thyroid hormones by the thyroid gland. The tropic hormones secreted by the hypothalamus are called *hypophysiotropic hormones* because they act on the hypophysis (pituitary gland). Also called *tropins*.

Tubular glands Exocrine glands whose pockets are tubular. Examples include sweat glands, intestinal glands, gastric glands, and bulbourethral glands.

Tumor angiogenesis factors (TAFs) Growth factors produced by normal and tumor cells. They stimulate the growth of new capillaries, organ regeneration, and wound healing.

Tumor necrosis factor (TNF) A small protein hormone secreted by macrophages. It stimulates the accumulation of leukocytes at sites of inflammation, activates inflammatory leukocytes to kill microbes, stimulates macrophages to produce IL-1, induces synthesis of colony-stimulating factors by endothelial cells and fibroblasts, exerts an interferonlike effect against viruses, and induces fever.

Tyrosine   An amino acid from which thyroid hormones, epinephrine, and norepinephrine are synthesized.

Up-regulation   A phenomenon in which there is an increase in the number of receptors in response to a deficiency of a hormone or neurotransmitter.

Urea   The major nitrogenous waste product of protein breakdown and amino acid catabolism. It is excreted by the kidneys in urine.

Vasopressin   *See* Antidiuretic hormone.

Vesicle   A small bladder or sac containing liquid.

Vitamin D   *See* Calcitriol.

Water-insoluble hormones   Steroid hormones and thyroid hormones.

Water-soluble hormones   Peptides, proteins, and catecholamines (epinephrine and norepinephrine).

Zona fasciculata   The middle layer of the adrenal cortex that secretes the hormone cortisol.

Zona glomerulosa   The outer layer of the adrenal cortex that secretes the hormone aldosterone.

Zona reticularis   The inner layer of the adrenal cortex that secretes small quantities of sex hormones.

Bibliography

Crapo, Lawrence.　*Hormones : The Messengers of Life.*
New York : W. H. Freeman, 1985.

Dorland, William Alexander.　*Dorland's Illustrated Medical Dictionary,* 27th ed.
Philadelphia : W. B. Saunders, 1988.

Ganong, William F.　*Review of Medical Physiology,* 15th ed.
Norwalk, Connecticut : Appleton & Lange, 1991.

Junqueira, L. Carlos, Jose Carneiro, and Robert O. Kelley.　*Basic Histology,* 6th ed.
Norwalk, Connecticut : Appleton & Lange, 1989.

Kapit, Wynn and Lawrence M. Elson.　*The Anatomy Coloring Book.*
New York : Harper & Row, 1977.

Melloni, B. J., Ida Dox, and Gilbert Eisner.　*Melloni's Illustrated Medical Dictionary,* 2nd ed.
Baltimore : Williams & Wilkins, 1985.

Tortora, Gerard J. and Sandra Reynolds Grabowski.　*Principles of Anatomy and Physiology,* 7th ed.
New York : HarperCollins, 1993.

Vander, Arthur J., James H. Sherman, and Dorothy S. Luciano.　*Human Physiology,* 5th ed.
New York : McGraw-Hill, 1990.